"I have been struggling with being overweight most of my life. Food has been my comfort. I heard about Carol's program through my job. Starting it was one of the best things I have ever done for myself. I have done many different weight-management programs in the past. A few worked at getting pounds off, but none kept the weight off. Carol's program was different from all the other programs I tried.

Now, four months later and twenty-five pounds lighter, I feel great. I have gone down almost two sizes in my clothes and both my blood pressure and cholesterol count have dropped to normal levels. I no longer experience daily headaches and I have lots more energy. I owe all this to Carol for creating this program and for supporting me in my goal to change my life."

—K.U.

"It is with great appreciation that I write this letter regarding Carol Simontacchi's weight program. With the program I began to feel better, and the weight, inches, and fat came off on a fairly regular basis. After three months on the program I was within ten pounds of my goal.

I can't even remember being hungry. The luscious recipes Carol provided brought the joy back into cooking. It was fun to create new flavors I hadn't tasted before.

My total weight loss with this program was forty pounds. I feel so much better about the way I look and am not ashamed to be seen any longer. It's so much fun."

—Mary

"I had hopes, but was not totally convinced that at age sixty-three I could lose my unwanted weight. Two years earlier I had been diagnosed with rheumatoid arthritis and the medication and lack of exercise had caused a weight gain of thirty-five pounds. In five months I lost thirty pounds and my blood pressure and cholesterol had dropped. I don't think of this program as a 'diet,' but as a life-time change in my eating habits."

—P.E.

"Joining Carol's program is one of the best things I have ever done for myself."

—Kathy

"The most important things I learned on Carol's program were how to take care of myself and live healthy for the rest of my life."

—Maggie

"When I started I was 198 pounds. Now I am 168 pounds and still losing weight. I get compliments regularly from those who know me on how great I look. I have gone from a full size eighteen to a size twelve.

To my enjoyment, Carol has introduced me to a whole new way of eating that satisfies my hunger and meets my nutritional needs, with even a few 'goodies' thrown in. Within the first week of my new food plan, I not only saw immediate weight loss, but I experienced a whole new satisfied feeling.

It is now second nature to me to make food selections that agree with my body's metabolism. If I listen to how my body responds to the right kind of food, I know I'm guaranteed success. In my mind there are very few people who would not be totally successful on this program. It is a lifestyle change that can and will make you fat-free for life! Thank you, Carol!"

—J.H.

"I am grateful to Carol for this weight-loss program. It's an absolute blessing to me. Because of her, my life has permanently changed for the better.

At the beginning of this program, I followed all the instructions and joyously made the delicious recipes, but the weight wasn't coming off and all the old feelings came plummeting back. But with Carol's constant encouragement, support, and belief in me, I realized it wasn't my fault. After finding out I had low thyroid and adrenal functions, and getting the doctor's care I needed, the weight came tumbling down!

I have lost thirty-five pounds, gone down three sizes, and my energy level has greatly increased. I feel so good about myself."

—S.L.

"I gave my clothes to my dad and laughed. I can cheat once in a while and not feel guilty. I'll never gain the weight back again because I'm in control."

—John

"After going through so many weight-loss programs and not being able to lose weight, I felt that I didn't even want to live. I was so depressed. Thank you, Carol! I've lost over thirty-five pounds and feel wonderful!"

—Jane M.

"This was the easiest weight-loss program I've ever gone on. Even though I can't cook, I found I could follow these recipes. Even my friends can't believe I'm actually making gourmet diet food!"

—Sandra

"If anybody tells you they can't succeed on this program, they haven't tried! Carol's program is so easy, it makes so much sense, and my body feels so good on it that there is no excuse for failure. I will never go back to my old way of eating."

—Jane S.

"After just six weeks on this program, my shoes are falling off my feet and I'm already out of my clothes. I just bought new sneakers and already they are too big for me. Help! I need new clothes!"

—Pat

"Carol, thank you so much for writing this book. I've been using your program now for over a year and have lost over 100 pounds. My only question is, can you write some more recipes? This is the best food I've ever eaten."

—Anne

"My friends keep saying, 'How did you lose all that weight?' But I promised not to share the recipes with anyone until the book came out. Please, Carol . . . I can't hold them off much longer! We need this book!"

—Judy

"Four weeks ago I gave up sugar. It wasn't even hard for me. There have been some days where something is missing and I recognize it's not that 'thought craving' but something is missing and I wind up eating something I shouldn't be eating. But I've not gone back to sugar! I have been *to six birthday parties, a wedding shower, a baby shower, a wedding, and four Women's Bible Studies. I've served four times, and I haven't even licked a finger. It's a miracle!"*

—Sally

"You come to a moment in time where you realize that the decision to lose weight is there, and it is a mental decision. It is not 'Well, some-day . . .' Today is the day I start! And that's it! You don't look back!"

—Esther

"After discussing my client's needs with her physician, I put her on a safe, well-balanced herbal formula to stimulate thermogenesis, and sat back nervously to wait. If this failed, I dreaded talking with her again. I expected her to call but the phone didn't ring, so after waiting for about six weeks, I picked up the telephone to call her. 'I only call when I'm up-set,' she explained. 'So far I have lost thirty-five pounds, I feel fabu-lous—better than I have in years—and the weight is still dropping. I'll be down to my ideal weight by Christmas. I'm following your diet rec-ommendations, too!' I frankly didn't have anything to say. 'Oh, and by the way,' she said. 'Thank you.' You're welcome. . . ."

—Carol Simontacchi

Your Fat
Is Not
Your
Fault

Your Fat Is Not Your Fault

Overcome Your Body's Resistance to Permanent Weight Loss

CAROL SIMONTACCHI, C.C.N., M.S.

Delicious, easy gourmet recipes by chef MARGARET WEST

Jeremy P. Tarcher/Putnam
a member of
Penguin Putnam Inc.
New York

An important note: This book is not intended as a substitute for the medical recommendations of physicians or other health-care providers. Rather, it is intended to offer information to help the reader cooperate with physicians and health professionals in a mutual quest for optimum well-being.

The publisher and the author are not responsible for any goods and/or services offered or referred to in this book and expressly disclaim all liability in connection with the fulfillment of orders for any such goods and/or services and for any damage, loss, or expense to person or property arising out of or relating to them.

Book design by Mauna Eichner

acknowledgments

This book could not have been written without the valuable experience my clients offer. I am deeply grateful for their encouragement and their excitement about being included in the project! It has been so interesting, so *much fun* getting to know all of them and working through their special needs.

I am also deeply grateful to Dr. Barry Sears for the opportunity to work with him. His insight into the insulin/glucagon role in weight loss and health management has been an invaluable part of my own ongoing training. Not only did he teach me the concepts of dietary balance, he pointed the way for me to obtain information from other sources and has been a continual source of information.

And, of course, this book would have been so much more difficult to read if it weren't for Traci Mullins, Deena Davis, and the rest of the Piñon editorial staff. They shuffled the pieces of my manuscript around, and when they put it back together again, it was a better book. I'm willing to admit that freely, now that I've gotten over the agony of it!

And, of course, my final thanks go to the staff at Health Haus and the Natural Physician Center. You've been willing to let me shut myself in my office and peck away at the computer, believing that someday both I and a book would emerge. Your faith was not in vain. Thank you for giving me the time and space to do what I've wanted to do for a long time. You are a great team!

*This book is dedicated to the most
supportive husband in the world. Bob,
you are my "kite string." With you,
I can fly higher and farther than
I ever dreamed possible.*

*And to my four beautiful daughters.
Girls, thank you for loving me,
each in your own unique way.
You are the joy of my life.*

*And most of all, to my
Heavenly Father, who daily fills me
with more grace and health than
I have ever deserved.*

contents

foreword

Carol presents a unique perspective for the average American who continues to struggle with weight loss. As an owner of a very successful chain of health food stores in the Northwest, she has an understanding of the desires of the individual who is seeking a "magic pill" to reduce excess body fat. Even with her extraordinary knowledge of nutritional supplements, she realized the complete answer was never going to be found in some bottle, and that even the best supplementation program had to be combined with an appropriate dietary plan. But which one?

I had the pleasure to meet Carol some eight years ago as I was developing the fundamental theories of using diet to control insulin. Carol quickly realized that a dietary program based on insulin control coupled with appropriate nutritional supplementation finally offered a comprehensive strategy to what has become an epidemic problem in America: obesity. In this book, Carol skillfully combines her knowledge of nutrition, an academic understanding of the hormonal aspects of diet, and her commitment as an educator. The end result is an informative and easy-to-follow dietary strategy to make permanent weight loss a reality.

BARRY SEARS, PH.D.

author of *The Zone* and *Mastering the Zone*

The
Fattening
of
America

Remember the old saying "Animals sweat; men perspire; women glow"? Forget it. If you're a nineties kind of person, male or female, you sweat . . . and you boast about it. ✂ Today fitness is big business. Health clubs are one of the hottest business opportunities, followed closely by weight-loss centers, diet books, and workout wear. And what about the way we eat? Low-fat or fat-free, artificially sweetened, high fiber, low cholesterol, vegetarian, low salt, whole grain . . . take your pick. If it sounds healthy, it's in.

But consider this: With all the interest in healthy food and a healthy lifestyle, why is America so fat? And why are we getting fatter every year?

Each spring, weight-loss books proliferate on bookstore and supermarket shelves like crabgrass spreading through a lawn. Drug companies challenge expensive research staffs to synthesize magic pills that promise to melt the fat off your hips without asking for dietary sacrifices. Madison Avenue admonishes us: "Just do it!" So we pull out our credit cards for jogging shoes, hiking shoes, biking shoes, aerobic shoes, tennis shoes, walking shoes, boxing shoes—not to mention high-heeled sneakers. We buy Cardioglides, Healthriders, treadmills, rowing machines, ankle weights, wrist weights, stationary bikes, barbells, Nordic-Tracks, Thighmasters and Buttmasters. We buy video workout tapes that promise eight-minute abs and eight-minute buns and turn our TV rooms into in-home health clubs.

Sweat is like a sacred ointment with which we seek absolution from our dietary sins, and we feel guilty if we don't anoint ourselves every morning.

For all this effort we're still fat. Over 51 percent of Americans are overweight, and these percentages are increasing every year.[1] Approximately 12.5 million Americans are severely overweight, and of these, 8.4 million are morbidly obese—over 140 percent of their ideal weight.

The middle of America (pardon the pun) seems to be increasing the fastest, with the highest incidence of obesity in the Midwest (particularly in Wisconsin and Indiana) and the lowest in the West (particularly in New Mexico).[2]

> *"I dress to hide myself. Large clothes, drapey clothes, nothing tucked in. Nothing that is real binding, nothing that shows the tummy rolls."*
>
> **NATALIE**

Obesity used to be an adult problem—that "middle-aged spread" we laughed about. It was the guy who complained of his "furniture problem" (his chest sinking into his drawers) or the dumpy dowager or the frumpy middle-aged mom. Obesity is no longer just an adult problem. According to recent statistics, obesity among our younger generation has more than doubled in the past decade, up to 11 percent from just 5 percent in our six- to seventeen-year-old children. More than 22 percent of all children under the age of eighteen are "potentially overweight."[3] Currently, 25 percent of American kids are at risk for the adult consequences of being overweight.[4] Yes, obesity is now a pediatric condition with consequences that reach far into adulthood.

Some parents view the weight challenges of their chubby youngsters as a problem they'll outgrow. But according to the American Institute of Nutrition, this simply isn't the pattern. Most overweight children grow up to be overweight adults, with eating habits and weight challenges so firmly ingrained in their physiques that it becomes next to impossible to normalize their weight without extraordinary effort.

The health consequences of this pattern are bringing the health-care system of the richest nation in the world to its knees. Fat is a very serious problem in this country—economically, medically, and socially.[5] The weight-loss industry is a $33 billion a year industry, with a failure rate of over 95 percent.[6]

This is not to say that all dietary failure is the result of a poor diet plan. Dieters aren't exactly known for willing compliance with restrictive eating regimens. In fact, two of my recent clients dropped out of the program just because they were "tired of being told what to eat. . . ." And one client wouldn't set aside time in his schedule to plan and prepare healthy meals, even when he knew that by doing so his former svelte waistline would reappear.

Yet the truth remains that obesity costs the United States over $40 billion a year—more than 5 percent of all illness-related costs in our society—and the numbers continue to rise.[7]

What, in the age of Diet Pepsi, Olestra, fat-free potato chips, sparkling mineral water, frozen Weight Watchers and Jenny Craig entrées, Ultra Slim-Fast, and pocket calorie counters, is making our kids and adults overweight? We're eating fewer calories than we've ever eaten, other than in famine conditions (total energy intake in the United States has decreased by 10 percent since 1900), yet obesity has more than doubled in the same period of time. The issues of obesity and even minor weight challenges may be much more complex than most people think.

For some, dieting is a lifestyle. It's just what they do, sort of like a vocation or a hobby. But for many others, their dress or pant size is a nightmare that haunts them every time they step outside the front door, every time they go shopping for clothes or food, every time they sit down in a nice restaurant to eat, every time they invite someone over for coffee. Weight has taken a huge toll on their mental, physical, social, and spiritual health. They would do literally anything to stop the pain.

If you're one of these people, if you really have tried every diet, you really have complied with doctors' orders, you really are willing to do whatever it takes to regain control over your waistline, this book may unlock the mystery of why maintaining your desired weight seems like an impossible task. This book is written for every man or woman who has ever sincerely tried to lose the weight but lost the battle.

These are the individuals who suffer from what I call "stubborn obesity." These are the ones who struggle with female hormones, adrenal exhaustion, or sluggish thyroid, or who just can't find a reasonable explanation for why they remain fat on the same number of calories or low-fat diet their skinny neighbors eat. Most of all, this book is written for every man and woman who just wants to end the weight struggle and look *and feel* good again!

fighting cultural prejudice

It would be one thing, from a health perspective, if weight were a reliable indicator of health. But it isn't. Some of the unhealthiest people I know are very thin, and some of the healthiest people I know sport at least twenty or more "extra" pounds. Some of my thin friends have the most terrible eating habits, consuming enormous quantities of the worst that the junk food industry offers. They smoke cigarettes, drink alcohol, and engage in other high-risk behaviors. In fact, they *can't* gain weight because their bodies are struggling just to stay alive. And some of my heavier friends watch their diets with the vigilance of a mother eagle, and their faces glow with an *inner* health their thin friends should envy. No, the scale is not always a measure of health status.

But we aren't convinced. We cover up our weight with stylish clothes, hats, long hair, baggy pants, or any other device we hope will take the emphasis off our expanding waistlines, because we know we'll be harshly judged if it shows.

An article in the *Executive Health Report* spoke eloquently on the pain of being overweight, stating that "obese persons in the United States are subject to 'intense prejudice and discrimination,' beginning early in childhood and lasting for life."[8]

*"If you tell me that I cannot
have that, that I cannot ever
have that, it's the end."*
ETTA

How did weight get to be such an emotional issue? When we look back just a few centuries into the works of some of the great artists, we see a concept of beauty that would do well for us today. Round-faced, round-bodied women. Full-chested men who stuck out hefty anteriors with a savoir faire that only a society that boasts of bigness could appreciate. Most of the artists whose works have endured through the ages featured women carrying at least twenty-five to thirty pounds more than we consider ideal. As a matter of fact, the women in Greek sculpture tended to be just a little hippy, according to our taste. But in those times, portliness was associated with prosperity. The woman or man whose figure was more round than angular could afford more and better food. Body shape wasn't so much a fashion statement as a barometer of status.

Just which fashion designer decided for the rest of the world that slim is in and plump is dumpy? We can't be sure who first birthed the idea that "you can't be too rich or too thin," but let's accept our share of the responsibility. We've all said it, although if we thought about it for longer than a second or two, we'd see the utter foolishness of it. I don't know if one can be too rich but I do know we can be too thin.

Body size and shape is such a complicated issue for us, especially if weight is indeed a health challenge and not just some vain obsession to lose five pounds. But even if our weight is a health issue and not a case of vanity, it still carries emotional and spiritual baggage unlike any other health condition. If we develop gallstones or a lung disease, if our knees go bad, or some other "invisible" ailment overtakes us, we can simply hide it or accommodate it and go on with our lives. We certainly don't feel shame or disgust.

Weight is different. We shake our fists at the scales. We whimper about our clothing size. We suck in our gut to try to conform to the image we've cast in our minds. In short, we do everything we can to look like what we are not and be what we will never be—the reincarnation of Twiggy or Arnold Schwarzenegger. This wouldn't be so painful if our culture didn't agree with us. Just try to accept the few extra pounds that sculpt your figure, and buy a size larger, and you invite the scorn of every passerby who weighs just a little less.

One author wrote:

> Numerous studies have documented the stigmatization of obese persons in more areas of social functioning. Children as young as six years describe obese children as "lazy, dirty, stupid, ugly, cheats, and liars." As they grow older, obese persons find they are less likely to be admitted to prestigious schools, to enter desirable professions, to receive equal pay for their work and respectful treatment by their doctors. Of all conditions for which a person may be stigmatized in our culture, the stigmatized overweight may be the most debilitating. . . . Furthermore, the stigma of overweight has two aspects: stigmatization of the appearance of the body and the stigmatization of the character of the person for the moral failure of not controlling one's weight.[9]

Some years ago I stepped out of a radio station with a well-known talk show host. With her frosted hair, her size-10 pantsuit, and her polished nails, she looked as if she had stepped right off Rodeo Drive. As we pushed open the door, two overweight women walked by. My host took one look at them and said, "Isn't that disgusting? Just look at them! Why don't they do something about that?"

My heart went out to those two women. After working with obese people over the years and watching their frustration explode into fury at bodies that simply won't cooperate with the very best efforts, I surmised that these women possibly had done everything they knew to keep the scale under control, but with little success.

> *"I did what was politically correct and I still gained weight."*
> ETTA

Obesity is seldom a case of overindulgence. It may simply be that an obese person's body works differently from a "normal" person's body, and the obese person hasn't been taught how to compensate for his or her own unique health needs.

Unfortunately, many doctors who should know better feel free to chastise their obese patients as they would a willful child. Pat spoke of her humiliation: "I don't go to the doctor my family uses because he's into: 'It's your fault.'" I asked Pat if she felt like an overweight object with her doctor. She grimaced and replied, "They give you that little look that says, 'How could you?' They make you feel uncomfortable."

Samantha nearly burst into tears when we discussed her doctor visits. "One time I had an inner ear infection and went to see the doctor four times before he would actually look at my ear," she said. "When I finally crawled in (I had lost my equilibrium), he decided it wasn't my weight after all. One doctor tweaked my knee and said, '*When* are you going to do something about this?' I hadn't even asked him about weight; I went in for something else."

Samantha then talked about the doctors who performed her stomach bypass surgery. "When they couldn't figure out why I regained the weight [after the surgery], they tried to talk me into intestinal bypass surgery, and I refused. I found out later that many people die from that surgery, but the doctors don't care. We're just fat people. We really don't matter to them."

Whether or not Samantha's perception is a true reflection of the medical community's attitude is irrelevant; her experience is a thread running through discussions I have with almost all of my obese clients. Their doctors don't show compassion; they show judgment.

One author, writing in the *Medical World News,* said that "many doctors in the health field are insensitive to fat people since it is very hard to help them. They lose their empathy and compassion which grows out of the thought from days past where obesity was viewed as an addiction or 'gluttony.' . . . Physicians need to be more understanding. . . ."[10]

Those of us who are not obese can't even imagine this type of demeaning attitude from professionals we're told to trust. But let's face it: Our culture discriminates against fat people in their work, in their social lives, in their medical treatment, in every part of their lives.

Pat told of one incident so casually that I almost didn't catch the tears in her voice as she related it. "One time someone harassed me going down the highway. These two teenagers cut me off and stopped in the middle of the highway. And I had my son in the car."

"Did you feel that was because of how you look?" I asked.

She nodded her head. "Oh, yes. They were making comments and teasing me."

but i want to be skinny!

It's doubtful that you or I can do anything about society's discrimination against overweight people. We can't change the world. And this prejudicial attitude is likely to worsen as more and more companies get involved in the fitness revolution sweeping the country. As advertising campaign megabucks continue to flow for fitness equipment, gyms, sneakers, diet drinks, and weight-loss pills, we're going to feel increasing pressure to conform to what the world thinks is the ideal weight for each of us.

We can, however, change our own attitudes about our weight. It isn't that the fitness revolution is negative; we all should be pursuing optimum health, whatever that means for each of us. And we need all the help we can get because those fitness ads are sandwiched between the junk food commercials. Talk about a schizophrenic media culture! On the one hand we're encouraged to grease our wheels at the local fast-food outlet and then we're challenged to unload that truckload of fat by working up a sweat on the latest exercise equipment.

your fat is not your fault

Because obesity is such a personal and deeply painful condition, and can be so difficult to resolve, it has taken on burdensome and often inappropriate psychological and spiritual dimensions. Dr. Judi Hollis, Ph.D., wrote in her book, *Fat and Furious*, that she never met a fat person who wasn't full of anger and depressed. I hope that isn't true. I hope most people with a weight problem see it for what it really is—a physical disability that can be resolved. But I fear Dr. Hollis may be right.

For many, the frustrating cycle of lose it/gain it/lose it/gain it has worn down their emotional and spiritual defenses, leaving them easy prey to the ultimate victimizer—self-loathing. Those who categorize weight challenges as spiritual weakness can load on more guilt and shame than we can bear, even if we're spiritually strong. The most casual, button-pushing phrases do it to us: "If you just prayed a little more"; "You just need a little faith"; "Don't think about yourself and food so much . . . get your mind on something other than your stomach." As if you could simply *think* your fat away.

One famous mental health clinic finds a psychological base in a person's weight gain. They call it "taking out frustrations in life with a knife and fork . . ."[11] But if frustrations in life cause obesity, why don't we all weigh 400 pounds? Do thin people ever use food as comfort? Yes, of course. At times, we all eat inappropriately. When you consider the abuse society piles onto overweight people and the inner shame aroused when we encounter our expanding images in the mirror, one would think that obese people are the most psychologically and spiritually unhealthy people in the world!

Let's get this straight right from the beginning: Your eating habits may not be the best in the world, and perhaps you do eat too much junk food. Maybe you're one of those Mr. or Ms. Average Americans who drinks more soft drinks than water and eats most of your meals out of a box. And maybe you could include a few more fresh fruits and vegetables in your diet every day. But the reality is that your eating habits are no worse than your skinny neighbor's, and you probably don't eat any more donuts or potato chips than your svelte spouse.

Many of us *do* need to confront the past, acknowledge the

hurt inflicted on us by significant people in our lives, and let God heal the hurt within us. But the fact that we are overweight does not necessarily mean we're mentally or emotionally or spiritually sick. Sometimes what seems to be a spiritual or emotional problem really is a physical problem. We simply haven't been taught how to eat to stay slim.

Let's put this topic into a perspective that will empower us with both physical and emotional health. The first issue we need to look at is the basic question "How much weight do I really have to lose?" Many of us have adopted society's idea of the perfect physique without ever consulting our own bodies! For years we've depended on the Metropolitan Life Insurance Company tables to judge whether or not we are overweight. These tables have undergone several revisions since they were first published in 1942, but the original tables were composed as an attempt to assign the relative risk factor for death or to determine at which height/weight ratio longevity was increased. The tables had nothing to do with health or even the proportion of lean tissue to fat tissue.

During World War II a Navy physician named Behnke illustrated the shortcoming of the tables by hydrostatic weighing of football players who were "overweight" simply because their bodies were excessively muscular. This excited an interest in studying the composition of the human body, and this field is still being studied exhaustively today.[12]

While many practitioners now believe those tables are overly conservative in their estimate of ideal weight, we still try to get our measuring devices to align with the figures in those tables and embark on desperate attempts to lose weight when our own bodies are screaming, "I feel good weighing just what I weigh now!"

Judy found that instead of needing to lose forty-five pounds, she looked great just losing thirty-five pounds. She looked good at a weight of 160. Marina found that her ideal weight hovered around 155 and fluctuated about five pounds around that range. Bill feels great at 200 pounds, even though he *thinks* he should weigh about 175. Maybe the body really does know best.

I had to learn this lesson along with my clients. I danced through my twenties and early thirties in a size 10 dress, weighing 137 pounds at 5 feet 9 inches. I was thin and proud of it! But when I married my husband, he had little appreciation for the shape of his bony bride. So he secretly decided to fatten me up!

I had no idea what was happening, because I had *never* experienced weight gain other than a pound or so around menses. Within just a few months of being lavishly courted by this affectionate man, I had gained enough weight to burst the seams on all my clothes. We went on a wild shopping spree for size-14 clothes! He frankly enjoys hugging a body that feels softer and rounder than the bag of bones he married.

While I'm definitely *not* advocating letting someone else tell us how to look or what size we should be (we alone know when our bodies feel good), this experience gave me a different perspective on beauty.

I have never again weighed 135 pounds. My body is happy at 160. I work hard to stay in shape and keep this middle-aged body physically fit, but I have no illusions about shopping the size-10 rack at Nordstrom's. I've learned how to dress beautifully in a size 12 or even a size 14.

This is the type of body acceptance we all can enjoy. What do you think is your ideal weight? Is that where your body feels and looks good? Can you be happy at that weight? Is it realistic to expect the same shape at the age of forty-five that you enjoyed (prechildren) at twenty-five? If a fifty-year-old man starts putting in time at the local gym, pumping iron with the younger guys, can he ever look like the football star he was in his early twenties? Probably not. Shapes change. Weights change. Body fat percentages change. And just recognizing that our bodies are changing and that change is healthy for us can be deliciously liberating to even the most weight-conscious among us.

Obesity is a complex issue that can be resolved for about 80 percent of the people who use the techniques I will describe in this book. The remaining 20 percent who struggle with "stubborn obesity" may continue to be challenged by their weight at every step. They may eventually lose it with enormous effort or they simply may not be able to lose it no matter what they do. And these are the people who need to learn to love themselves and accept their bodies for what they are, with the same grace they offer themselves if they are suffering from an ulcer, heart disease, or weak ankles.

> "Quite frankly, fat people are going to go to heaven just like skinny people. It's just as much a sin for a guy to consume two boxes of Twinkies."
> **MIKE**

If you are carrying around 20—or 120—pounds of guilt, lay it aside right now. You aren't a weak-willed ninny. You probably aren't a closet eater. Your eating habits may be no worse than those of your spouse, your sister, your friend, or your neighbor who never gains a pound on twice the food consumption. You really can put on five pounds from just one chocolate chip cookie or a handful of potato chips. Your body refuses to lose weight on your lettuce-leaf-and-carrot-stick diet, no matter how faithfully you follow it. And you aren't just hiding behind your fat to avoid emotional issues. Your body is different. It doesn't work the way it's supposed to.

Your body is stubbornly resisting weight loss because you haven't been taught how to eat, how to stop dieting, and how to use food to build vibrant health. Dieting has not worked for you because *it cannot work for you*. The dieting style of the eighties and nineties is genetically and biologically wrong for us, no matter how many weight-loss magazine articles and books are written about how to do it their way. It won't work—ever.

The message in this book isn't a plan that advocates starvation or asceticism. I share specific principles about weight and weight loss that you may never have understood before. In this book you will learn a new way to eat, and hopefully end your "dieting" days forever.

PRINCIPLES TO LIVE (AND LOSE) BY

Let's look at some of these principles, one at a time:

Principle #1 If you are overweight now or have been overweight in the past, you are permanently overweight. Period. You will never lose your tendency to be fat, no matter what you do. Yes, that is a depressing message, but there are two important biological reasons for this principle: 1) you have too many fat cells, and 2) these cells always want to be filled up with fat.

If overeating resulted in weight gain at some time in your life, or if you inherited a predisposition toward obesity, your body has generated too many fat cells, and these cells will not disappear no matter how disciplined you may be or how much weight you lose. Every one of those greedy little fat cells is there to stay. And just like savings banks that get nervous when they run short of money, fat cells get nervous when they run short of fat. They aren't stable unless their storage tanks are filled up. So even if you lose excess weight, if you then resume old eating patterns, those fat cells will suck up the excess calories or carbohydrates or fats and deposit them back in the tank. Fat cells are genetically programmed to increase their stores, and there is no way you can change that.

Therefore, the only way to keep your weight stable after you have suffered from obesity is to alter the way you eat so that you don't give your fat cells the opportunity to fulfill their genetic destiny. While you can't "cure" obesity in the truest sense of the word, you don't have to be fat. Fortunately, it isn't even that hard to be slim. You just have to know how to do it, and I'll teach you how in the pages of this book.

Principle #2 Almost everything you read in the mainstream media about nutrition and diets is wrong. Guaranteed. The politically correct diets of the eighties and nineties are guaranteed to make you fatter. If you don't believe that, consider how many weight-loss books, products, and programs are sold every year. Given all this money and attention devoted to losing weight, are we getting slimmer? Are we getting healthier?

Consider how many diets you've tried. Is it getting easier for you take the weight off and keep it off? Absolutely not. That's why you're reading this book.

Around 95 percent of dieters regain their weight, often gaining more weight than when they started. They continue to diet over and over again, sometimes losing hundreds of pounds over the course of a lifetime, only to gain it all back. If you want to lose weight permanently, you're going to have to do something different! You're going to have to stop dieting and learn how to eat and how to live.

Listen closely: YOU MUST NEVER GO ON A DIET AGAIN! It will ruin your health and make you fat!

Principle #3 It is possible to lose weight, feel great while doing it, and keep it off permanently.

This is the overriding message of this book. I will teach you why you have gained weight in the first place so that you can avoid pitfalls in the future. I will coach you on how to lose weight and maintain the loss. It's not going to be as difficult as you think. You won't have to choke down tasteless, cardboard-y, packaged foods. You won't have to go on drugs or have body parts stapled together. Instead, I'll teach you how to alter the way you look at food and how to adopt a new way of eating—forever.

The answer to lifelong weight management is restoring "balance" to your body. I'll tell you exactly what balance means, because the issues are much more complicated than the foods you choose to arrange on your dinner plate. You will see how a balanced endocrine system—especially a well-functioning pancreas—is critical to achieving a healthy weight. You'll find that dietary balance is achieved only by balancing the proteins, carbohydrates, and fats in your diet, not by going on some faddish food plan.

You must stop eating "diet" food and start eating real food, in the proper balance. Then you can make weight maintenance a permanent way of life and health.

how to use this book

Read through every page of this book before you try to put any of the principles into practice. Thoroughly understand each principle before you move on to the next. Read through the recipes (I'll warn you, they're tempting!). Start seeing yourself in these pages and plan how you'll structure your own program of weight maintenance.

Share this new eating plan with your physician and make sure you are physically able to make these changes in your diet. Discuss the various issues we raise with your health care practitioner. You'll especially want him or her to check the health of your kidneys, your endocrine system, your digestion, and your heart.

You'll need to include a gentle exercise program several times a week, so choose an exercise you really enjoy and mark it as a top-priority appointment on your calendar.

After you've familiarized yourself with how to build your whole-body health, put together your personalized program. Try to get your family involved. Let them know that as you get healthier, they will too. They'll enjoy eating these new foods with you. If possible, get someone to watch over you, to encourage you, to hold you to your commitment. You'll find accountability to be an important part of your long-term success.

Above all, don't think that this is just a summer or winter project—that when you've lost your weight and are feeling good, you'll resume your old way of eating and living. If you do, you'll regain every pound you worked so hard to lose—and a few extra for good measure.

Winning the weight game is not just a matter of following a program for a few weeks or months. Weight loss is not separate and apart from everything else you do in life. Weight *maintenance* is a lifestyle. It's the way you eat. Your body may respond to food differently from the bodies of normal-weight people, but that doesn't mean you're destined to be fat forever. It simply means you'll have to learn what satisfies your body and then do that consistently.

Now, let's get started. You're going to feel great!

Five Common Diet Strategies to Avoid

2

If you still think diets work, talk to Etta. She's tried them all. Weight Watchers . . . several times. Jenny Craig. A medically supervised fast. Calorie restriction. The only thing she figures she hasn't tried is stomach surgery. This is how Etta described her diet history.

When I'm in the diet mentality, I'm on a diet. When I go off the diet I go back to my regular lifestyle. Through all those years, I hadn't made a decision that this is a lifelong change. On the other programs I always had the idea that when I lost the weight, it would somehow stay off so I wouldn't have to follow the program anymore.

In the weight-loss clinics, I was hungry all the time. The only exception was the original Weight Watchers program where I was never hungry. Several years ago I did Weight Watchers for nine months and dropped ninety-six pounds. Then I went to San Francisco, visited Ghiradelli Square, had a hot fudge sundae, and that was the end. I never got back onto their eating plan!

I followed a medically supervised fast for six months, lost a lot of weight, and wasn't hungry. I didn't have to deal with food at all. I just drank the liquid stuff. I kept a list of foods I wanted to eat when I went off the fast, which set me up to fail. I had lost about 115 pounds and I was down to 200 pounds—for about fifteen minutes. But I had to start eating real food again. And that's when the weight all came back again.

Last year Etta decided to try a sensible weight-loss program, just one more time. She decided she was going to finally turn this thing around, so she followed the instructions of nearly every weight-loss professional (and every women's magazine) she could find and cut as much fat out of her diet as she could. She bought no-fat everything. She filled her plate with vegetables, pasta, and rice. She did it perfectly for six months—and put on thirty pounds. She followed the eating plan that was politically correct and gained weight!

Believe me, Etta knows how to follow a diet. So what's wrong? Why did the weight pile back on?

Those of us who have experimented with dieting for a while

have probably tried every weight-loss plan known to humankind—and failed. From the high protein to the high carbohydrate, from the low fat to the low calorie, from the liquid diet to Jenny Craig and Weight Watchers and TOPS. Even stomach bypass surgery. We did lose weight while we were on these programs, but as nearly all dieters find out sooner or later, it was nearly impossible to keep the weight off. Some studies show a 92 percent failure rate for *any type* of diet program! And each subsequent weight loss/weight gain cycle makes successive weight loss increasingly difficult.

The truth is simple: Diets don't work. The reason so many of us have failed to maintain weight is not that we lack willpower or self-control or can't follow instructions. It isn't simply that we eat too much. The reason is the dieting process itself. Diets lead to metabolic imbalances in our bodies that shape an internal environment which almost guarantees that we'll gain back the weight.

Let's examine the five most common diet strategies and why they fail. But first let's talk about the underlying problem that guarantees diet failure.

the low-calorie diet

The experts who make the simple connection that gluttony = obesity are wrong. Calories often have little to do with weight gain or loss. Just think about the people you know who can eat as much as they want and not gain an ounce. The whole concept of calorie counting when trying to lose weight is virtually a useless exercise. But the "experts" don't know that. One college textbook self-righteously proclaims:

> Weight gain or loss depends upon caloric intake and caloric use. If you consume more calories than you use, then you

will gain weight. Weight loss occurs when you use more calories than you consume. It is often said that the best form of exercise is to push yourself away from the table![1]

Let's think through the whole concept of calorie counting for a moment. The notion that overweighers are overeaters simply isn't supported by the facts. First of all, numerous studies have shown that overweight people eat statistically less food than normal or underweight people. But the issue goes even deeper than statistical averages into the topic of homeostasis—that is, *balance*. The healthy body can compensate for minor excesses and deficiencies of calories on a day-to-day, moment-to-moment basis. This compensatory mechanism is called *homeostasis*.

THE BODY'S NATURAL FOOD-BALANCING GAUGE

Homeostasis, the body's ability (among other things) to balance the amount of food eaten with the amount of food actually needed, is a function of the sympathetic nervous system over which we exert no conscious control. My dictionary likes a more complicated definition: "A state of physiological equilibrium produced by a balance of functions and of chemical composition within an organism."[2]

The word *homeostasis* is more easily understood by this explanation from *Nutrition and Diet Therapy:* "a tendency to stability in the internal environment of the organism; achieved by a system of control mechanisms activated by negative feedback."[3]

Simply stated, homeostasis is the body's way of normalizing itself, of adapting to a myriad of environmental conditions (both internal and external) to achieve balance in a changing environment. For example, though you may walk in and out of your air-conditioned home on a hot summer day, with temperatures fluctuating from 68 to 100 degrees in a matter of seconds, your body temperature remains relatively constant.

In the same way, your body makes infinite, second-by-second compensations to adjust for both excesses and deficiencies of calories every single day, at every single meal. Homeostatic mechanisms in the body allow us to consume an average amount of food each day without even considering caloric content. The body uses the calories for energy and, for the most part, maintains normal weight while doing it.

WHEN THE HOMEOSTATIC GAUGE IS BROKEN

Most of us tend to eat about the same amount of food at each meal (holidays excluded!). We eat until we're satisfied; then we stop eating. But just think about that for a moment. What makes us feel satisfied after a meal? Or, more important to the overweight individual who struggles with sub-optimal food choices, what keeps us eating long after our stomachs feel full, or nibbling on nonessentials when we aren't even hungry? It certainly isn't calories.

A person's caloric requirements are different from day to day or even from moment to moment. We require more calories when the ambient temperature drops or when our activity level increases, even if only temporarily. Caloric requirements drop when the sun comes out in the spring and summer or if we spend a few days in bed recovering from a bout of the flu.

If our bodies cannot adjust for these inconsistencies or tell us when to stop eating, how would we know just how many calories we need to maintain activity levels and maintain the same weight? Just how important are calories in maintaining homeostatic caloric balance, anyway?

> *"I wanted to do this program
> because it's one I've never
> tried before . . ."*
> **ESTHER**

Without homeostasis, weight control is impossible, even for those of us who are thin. Consider, for example, that it takes 3,500 excess calories to create one pound of fat. If we unwittingly consume just 100 excess calories per day (one piece of dry toast or a medium apple), we will gain one unwanted pound of body fat every thirty-five days. On the other hand, if we under-consume 100 calories every day, we will lose one pound every thirty-five days. Unless we take on the impossible task of adjusting our calorie count with every meal and snack, everyday, we will either gain or lose over one hundred pounds every ten years!

Part of the mechanism that achieves this balance is the normal body's ability to produce heat from food and to waste excess calories. For some people, those who struggle with excess weight, for example, this mechanism breaks down and the body loses the ability to "waste" calories.

An article published in *The Edell Health Letter* discussed the relationship between food intake and obesity. Researchers found that, overall, women who ate more food burned more calories—and stayed thinner in the process![4] Another article in *Nutrition Research Newsletter* stated:

> Several studies have shown that energy intake varies substantially among individuals, and that some "large eaters" do not become obese, while other "small eaters" seem to gain weight easily. . . .

> Dietary records showed that the large eaters consumed almost twice as much energy per kilogram of body weight. Despite this, they had lower body weights, lower body mass indexes, smaller anthropometric measurements of body fatness [sum of six skinfolds], and lower percent body fat than the small eaters did.[5]

It almost seems as though they're saying that if we *increase* the amount of food we're eating, we'll drop the excess weight. Wouldn't we love that! While we can't generalize the message to say that we simply need to eat more food if we want to shrink our waistlines, I think we can come to some obvious conclusions about these research findings. Something has gone very wrong.

What has gone wrong is that your homeostatic mechanism has broken down. Your body isn't processing the calories the way it needs to if you're going to maintain ideal weight. And this is what you need to fix. We'll discuss how to fix your homeostatic gauge in chapter 3 when we talk about BAT (brown adipose tissue). Meanwhile, if you usually arm yourself with a calorie counter guide before you sit down to eat dinner each night, throw it away.

side effects of low-calorie eating

OUT-OF-CONTROL EATING

Binge eating can be one result of following low-calorie diets. If your body feels like it's starving, it will demand food: "Give me chocolate chip cookies or give me death!" Binge eating episodes are often triggered in an attempt to normalize energy levels pulled down by a low-calorie diet.

One night after work, Sally decided she simply had to have a piece of strawberry rhubarb pie. She was in a hurry to get home. She didn't want to stop at a restaurant, so she stopped at the grocery store and purchased the pie she "needed." The clerk tossed a plastic fork and napkin into the bag (perhaps he saw the desperation in her eye?). Sally got back into the car and put the pie in the backseat for the long drive home. But the longer she drove, the more she thought about that pie in the box just behind her. She couldn't get it out of her mind.

At the next traffic light she reached back, opened the box, took a bite, and drove on. At the next traffic light she took another bite, then she pulled onto the freeway. No more traffic lights. Still that strawberry rhubarb pie beckoned.

It was pitch-dark and pouring down rain. Sally wanted to get home, but finally she couldn't stand the thought of that pie another moment. She pulled over to the side of the freeway, put on her emergency lights, and went to work on it. Before she pulled back onto the freeway and continued her trek home, she had eaten all but a small piece. She took the last sliver home and put it in the freezer. And when it was frozen solid, she finished it off with a cup of coffee!

Judy recalled how she woke up one Saturday, looked around the kitchen to see what there was to eat, and ate continuously for twelve hours straight. She ate bacon, bread, cookies, ice cream, sausages—anything that even resembled food—and she didn't even want it! She just ate it and didn't know why.

Binge eating, or Binge Eating Disorder (BED), is poorly understood in the scientific community. While some men indulge in binge eating, it is women who do it on a regular basis. In fact, three women for every two men are diagnosed with this disorder.[6] Some studies have cited that up to 46 percent of obese individuals enrolled in weight-reduction programs suffer from it,[7] and the incidence of this and other eating disorders is increasing.[8]

What is binge eating? According to the American Psychiatric Association, the following criteria must be present for a diagnosis of BED:

> Recurrent episodes of binge eating characterized by:
>
> 1.   Eating in a discrete period of time (in any two-hour period) an amount of food that is definitely larger than most people would eat during a similar period of time.
>
> 2.   A sense of lack of control during the episodes—a feeling that one can't stop eating or control what or how much one is eating.

During most binge-eating episodes, at least three of the following behavioral indicators of loss of control are present:

1.   Eating much more rapidly than usual.

2.   Eating until feeling uncomfortably full.

3.   Eating large amounts of food when not feeling physically hungry.

4.   Eating large amounts of food throughout the day with no planned meal times.

5.   Eating alone because of embarrassment over how much one is eating.

6.   Feeling disgusted with oneself, depressed, or guilty after overeating.

7.   Marked distress regarding binge eating.

8.   Binge-eating episodes occur, on average, at least twice a week for a six-month period.

9. Does not currently meet the criteria for bulimia nervosa or abuse medication (diet pills) in an attempt to avoid weight gain.[9]

If you have been "food deprived" (you have been dieting or eating too few calories), you are more likely to indulge in binge eating.[10]

A study of former prisoners of war may shed some light on why this is so. During World War II, researchers wanted to learn more about the effects of starvation. They recruited a number of young, healthy volunteers for their study who willingly went on a starvation diet and brought their weight down to 74 percent of what it should have been. They were literally starving to death in a laboratory! After researchers had achieved the weight-loss results they wanted, the volunteers were invited to bring their food consumption levels back to normal. Within a short period of time, these healthy men had regained the weight they had lost during the experiment.

Researchers noted one major change in their subjects. Now, when they sat down to a meal, they couldn't stop eating! They gorged beyond their physical limits! Something within their bodies had changed during that short period of starvation and they were no longer able to control how much food they ate. They continued to eat and eat and eat long after they were full.

A group of World War II prisoners underwent starvation during their incarceration period. After being released from captivity, researchers studied them to find the results of their terrible experience. There was overwhelming evidence that episodes of binge eating were common among these men who had suffered from starvation. In fact, the greater the degree of starvation, the greater the incidence of binge eating.[11]

> *"I would drive*
> *anywhere in the world for*
> *a maple bar . . ."*
> **SALLY**

Researchers did not say why this happened, only that evidence is clear that dieting (semistarvation) comes first, then binge eating.

Binge eating also may be an attempt by the body to normalize thyroid activity. Because BED patients have both a reduced metabolic rate and increased energy efficiency, and because the thyroid gland is the single most important controller of metabolic rate, the body may initiate overeating as a way to increase levels of thyroid hormone to stimulate the metabolic rate. In other words, binge eating may be a compensatory mechanism for a reduced thyroid function.[12]

Another compensatory mechanism may also be involved here. Binge eaters typically indulge in high-carbohydrate, sugary foods. A number of studies have shown that BED patients typically experience reduced levels of both serotonin and dopamine, both of which are calming neurotransmitters in the brain. The effect of inadequate levels of serotonin may lead to a reduced ability of the body to signal satiation, while low dopamine may lead to what one researcher called "hedonic responses to food."[13]

Carbohydrate or sugar intake can increase serotonin production in the brain, so one aspect of carbohydrate craving may be the body's way of increasing the production of this important neurotransmitter. Part of the body's own homeostatic function has turned self-destructive!

Because all the systems in the body are interdependent, alterations in many of the hormones and neurotransmitters may induce changes in the others and bring on many of the signs and symptoms of the BED patients. Changes in serotonin function can induce changes to adrenal hormones as well, causing a cascade of neurotransmitter/hormone dysfunction that produces a wide variety of symptoms, not the least of which is binge eating or other eating disorders.[14]

> *"One of the things that I said to myself is, 'What is it that I eat the most often? Taco Bell? McDonald's?' And then I'd lift my shirt up and I'd think, 'What good has it done me so far?'"*
>
> **MIKE**

As a clinical nutritionist, I have nearly always found that binge eating can be controlled more easily if my clients start eating a high-protein breakfast. When I put people on a soy-based protein drink spiked with flax oil for the benefits of the essential oils, and fresh fruit for flavor and carbohydrates, nearly all of them find both food cravings and the desire to indulge in binge eating greatly reduced.

Even if binge eating is not part of your personal profile but you find yourself indulging in the occasional impulsive snack simply because you "can't help yourself," eating a high-protein breakfast reduces the need for this type of unplanned eating that can stack on the pounds before you know it.[15]

EAT LESS, WEIGH MORE

The other major effect of a calorie-deprived diet is the inevitable weight gain. In a study of forty-nine obese women, the women were divided into two groups. One group maintained a 1,200 kcal diet each day throughout the fifty-two-week program, while the other group was treated (wrong word!) to a very low-calorie diet (420 kcal per day) for sixteen weeks, then brought back up to 1,200 kcal/day for the rest of the study period.

The women on the very low-calorie diet lost significantly more weight than the other women (21.45 kg vs. 11.86 kg) but they also regained a significant portion of that weight.[16]

Calories are relatively immaterial when it comes to weight loss. And nowhere is this more true than when discussing the high-carbohydrate/low-fat diet, the prevailing weight-loss paradigm of the nineties.

the high-carbohydrate diet

The high-carbohydrate diet is the politically correct diet of the last ten years, with literally hundreds of permutations centered on two main food groups: vegetables and grains, with small amounts of protein and minimal fats added as garnish. Sounds healthy, doesn't it? We're told by physicians, dietitians, nutritionists, and all sorts of authors that the vegetarian or the near-vegetarian diet is the perfect diet, and that we need to eat more fruits, vegetables, and grains. The recommendations are surrounded by scientific-sounding jargon.

In some respects, the proponents of this diet are right. We *do* need to eat more fruits and vegetables. After all, the typical American includes fewer than two servings of fruits and vegetables *combined* in his or her diet each day. The problem with predicating a weight-loss diet on a vegetable/grain-based diet, however, is that while it sounds scientific, it is also the wrong food plan for many people. The high-carbohydrate diet has some built-in flaws that guarantee eventual failure, particularly if your body is not genetically equipped to deal with all the sugars that high-carbohydrate foods produce.

Betty's story is a good example of what happens if your body is not meant for a high-carbohydrate diet.

> My mom was overweight and I have always had to be careful. In my country, Argentina, we eat a lot of wheat and beef. For breakfast we would have toast and maté (the Argentinean equivalent to coffee). Lunch usually consisted of noodles with a ground-beef sauce. We ate a lot of steak sandwiches (with bacon, cheese, lettuce, and tomatoes). A typical Argentinean family would have roast beef with vegetables and rice or noodles and a salad for dinner.
>
> My weight problem started when I went from a beef diet to a vegetarian diet. When I was eighteen, I went to college and gained about eighteen kilos (about forty pounds). Since then I have gone up and down.

Now forty-seven years old, Betty has seventy pounds to lose and has to be careful not to gain more. While a return to her beef-heavy childhood diet is not the answer for Betty, her strict vegetarian diet is not working either. She needs to learn how to balance her diet among protein, carbohydrates, and fats so that she can win the weight game she started playing over twenty years ago.

Before we look at why the balance of foods is so essential, let's explore the positive and negative sides of the high-carb diet.

THE PROS OF HIGH-CARB EATING

One of the gurus of the high-carbohydrate diet is John A. Mc-Dougall, medical doctor and author of several weight-loss books, including *The McDougall Program: 12 Days to Dynamic Health* and *The McDougall Plan*. Dr. McDougall's medical practice includes dietary approaches to treating disease. Dr. McDougall is well credentialed and acclaimed by religious leaders and medical doctors around the world.

Here is what Dr. McDougall suggests you eat for breakfast, lunch, and dinner:

Breakfast Suggestions:

Porridge, dry cereals with fruit juices and nut milks (a white beverage made from ground nuts and water), fruit sauces with toast or pancakes, baked sweet or white potatoes, rice and vegetables, fruits alone, fruit smoothies, or leftovers.

Lunch Suggestions:

Soup and bread, bean soups or chili served over pasta or other grain products, bean and grain soups, cold vegetable sandwiches, griddle cakes with beans or fruit sauces, raw vegetables with bean dip, fruit salad, raw fruits and vegetables.

Dinner Suggestions:

Day 1: Brown rice with vegetable stew and broiled zucchini

Day 2: Baked potatoes with mushroom gravy, and mixed peas and carrots

Day 3: Spaghetti noodles with tomato sauce, tossed salad with French tomato dressing

Day 4: White bean soup with whole-wheat bread and raw vegetables

Day 5: Brown rice with vegetable chop suey

Day 6: Baked sweet potatoes with cooked broccoli and mixed sprout salad

These menus simply burst with health and vitality! The emphasis on whole grains and vegetables sounds good ecologically, biologically, and politically, and you feel "righteous" just reading through them.

Another popular diet program is the "Fit For Life" plan in the book by the same name by Harvey and Marilyn Diamond. The concepts in their books are similar to McDougall's, but the Diamonds are not totally vegetarian. They recommend severely limiting both animal and vegetable proteins along with dietary fats, while significantly increasing carbohydrates. Another well-connected, well-published medical doctor, Dr. Neal Barnard, president of the Physicians' Committee for Responsible Medicine and leading authority on nutritional issues, bases his dietary suggestions on the same principles as the Diamonds but with a little more variety. Here is a sample of Dr. Barnard's protocol, based on the delicious, unlimited consumption of high-carbohydrate foods.[17]

Breakfast:

Cold cereal with soy milk, rice milk, or fruit juice with sliced banana and melon slices.

Lunch:

Black-bean burrito with bulgur and a salad (with no-fat dressing)

Dinner:

Roasted vegetables with tofu, risotto, squash, braised cabbage, and fruit for dessert

High-carbohydrate diets that are low in fat do have significant health benefits to offer, and while you will soon understand why I don't think they are appropriate for a weight-conscious public, I think we can learn something from them.

First of all, the emphasis on fresh fruits and vegetables is so important that this one factor alone makes these diets worthwhile for many people to consider. Because the average American eats so few fruits and vegetables and is suffering the health consequences of this dietary laziness, just scooping a few spoonfuls of vegetables onto the plate every evening makes a person feel better. The high-carb gurus have done the world a great service by calling our attention to the importance of eating food that at one time had roots deeply embedded in soil.

Second, as health experts have steered people away from eating rancid, toxic, processed fats, the resulting reduced serum cholesterol and triglyceride levels produce healthier hearts. Within the past few years, the broadcast and print media have pummeled the public with information on phytochemicals (natural chemicals within the vegetable world) that impart enormous health benefits. Much of the momentum behind this media interest comes from doctors who have seen the devastating consequences of indulging the palate with life-robbing nonfoods like potato chips, french fries, and diet soft drinks and they wish to educate the public away from the consequences that follow habitual consumption of them.

Now let's flip the coin over and look at the other side.

THE CONS OF HIGH-CARB EATING

Regardless of how it looks on paper, the high-carbohydrate diet program is wrong for nearly everyone, especially those unfortunate souls who struggle with obstinate excess weight.

Notice that I said *nearly* everyone. Our world is blessed with a staggering diversity of genetics and biochemical needs. No two people are alike, not even identical twins. While we can construct some generalizations (and we're going to do just that), no one diet is perfect for every person, no matter how righteous or healthy the diet, or how qualified the professional who offers it.

So why do so many people fail to maintain their ideal weight on a high-carb diet?

1. Most of the weight loss will be from loss of water and muscle tissue.

2. Because the diet is so low in calories, cellular fuel is underprovided, leading to loss of energy resources. In other words, you become tired.

3. The diet is difficult to sustain because of the hunger factor. You simply can't continue on a program forever if your stomach is growling. You'll either find yourself going off the diet completely or indulging in binge-eating episodes.

4. Blood sugar–regulating hormones become unbalanced.

5. Key nutrients are underprovided, such as essential amino acids and fatty acids, along with trace nutrients, such as certain vitamins and minerals. This leaves the body vulnerable to nutrient deficiencies, particularly if the diet is followed for a prolonged period of time.

To achieve and maintain weight loss throughout life, we must satisfy the body's very specific nutrient needs. We simply have to balance the diet. Why, then, do some people lose weight on a high-carbohydrate diet? Even if a diet is notoriously deficient in macronutrients, like protein or fat, or in micronutrients, like vitamins and minerals, people often feel better following it and lose lots of weight. Why?

Initially, they feel better because vegetables and fruits are

rich in essential minerals that fuel the enzymes and provide cellular energy. But beyond subjective feelings, the health of the
body cannot be maintained long-term unless all nutrients are being supplied on a daily basis. Protein is just one of those nutrients. And adequate protein is essential for maintaining lean
body tissue, primarily muscle tissue.

We have to ingest protein to preserve muscle tissue, which
comprises one-half or more of total body weight and includes the
vital organs. The most metabolically active tissue in the body is
what we call visceral tissue or internal organs, such as the heart,
liver, and kidneys. But protein is also used for such essential body
structures as hormones, neurotransmitters, enzymes, blood cells,
immune bodies, and more. These small but critical structures are
more important to life maintenance on a day-to-day basis than
muscle tissue. If the right elements are not present to synthesize
these structures, key functions in the body will not get done.

> *"I put my jeans on Monday
> and found they're way too
> big (after six weeks). But I'm
> falling out of my shoes! I
> just bought new shoes four
> weeks ago and they don't
> stay on my feet anymore!"*
>
> **BETH**

When we embark on a low-fat, low-protein, or low-*anything*
diet, weight loss is often achieved through the loss of muscle and
organ tissue. Muscle weighs more than fat, and it doesn't take
very much muscle loss to equal a substantial amount of weight

loss to the detriment of the organism involved. Muscle loss is *never* a good idea.

Rapid weight loss is our first clue that any loss we are enjoying is not from the loss of fat, but from the loss of water and muscle. While many overweight people sequester a little too much water, it's dangerous to reduce the water content of the body by more than about .5 percent (about three-fourths of a pound in an average-weight person).

If the diet remains protein deficient for very long, enough muscle tissue will be consumed or "cannibalized" to compromise the most important muscle of all—the heart. A diet that severely restricts proteins and fats can be fatal!

Another problem with high-carbohydrate diets is calorie deprivation. While eating nutrient-dense fruits and vegetables makes you feel better initially, unless you consume other macronutrients like proteins and fats, your internal energy stores are depleted, and within a short period of time you feel tired.

A study using rats showed that "animals fed a low-protein diet were hyperphagic" (they ate too much) and accumulated a greater amount of body fat. It seems that food deprivation or the low-calorie diet elevates a gene (the NPY gene) that stimulates food intake and increases body fat accumulation. The food-deprived rats were restricted in calorie intake by 50 percent. Interestingly, researchers restricted protein, not carbohydrates or fats. The authors of the study wrote:

> The major finding of the present study was that a low protein diet . . . seemed to be as effective as energy restriction in elevating NPY gene expression. Although protein restriction elevated NPY gene expression . . . we found no effect of either carbohydrate or fat restriction. . . . To more closely examine how protein restriction affected body weight, a body composition analysis was performed. Rats fed a protein-restricted diet had [about] 35% more body fat,

> both on a percent basis and on an absolute basis than rats
> fed the modified . . . diet. . . . Total body water was reduced
> to the same degree that body fat was elevated such that to-
> tal body weight was not altered. . . . The additional energy
> [calorie] intake of protein-restricted rats leads to a greater
> amount of body fat. . . .[18]

What we see here is that a high-carbohydrate/low-protein diet alters genetic ability to keep fat weight at a minimum. The *diet itself* causes the problem! The bottom line is that if you lose your weight and decide to go off the diet, you *must not* replace it with another form of the high-carbohydrate diet. If you do, your hard work will be rewarded by an even more powerful tendency to store even the smallest amount of excess calories on your hips and thighs. You are decidedly worse off than when you started.

If you're struggling with the high-carbohydrate diet, believing that you're dieting correctly but are failing miserably, don't despair. You're in the majority! The high-carbohydrate diet is not genetically right for you.

the low-fat diet

The low-fat diet is another politically correct, scientific-sounding, professionally marketed diet strategy that looks promising and works short-term but is bound to generate diet failure sooner or later. The frustrating problem with the doctrine of the low-fat diet is that it is partially correct: Americans *do* eat too much fat! They eat the *wrong* fats. Fat is calorie-dense, over nine calories per gram of fat as opposed to just over four calories per gram of carbohydrate or protein. If your aim is to drop calories, the likeliest target is dietary fat.

Losing weight isn't a simple matter of calorie or fat-gram

counting. The issues are much more complex, as we are beginning to see. We simply can't erase (or thoughtlessly reduce) one whole category of essential nutrients from our diet and expect our bodies to unload weight in appreciation. Fat is just one essential part of the diet. The term *essential fatty acids* is not a frivolous term because these necessary, life-conferring nutrients cannot be manufactured by the body; they must be obtained from the diet. In other words, fats are not the bad guys of the diet world; they are of primary importance!

Perhaps we can simplify this complex subject by looking at the facts.

1. Americans eat too much fat.

2. Americans eat the wrong kinds of fat.

3. People lose weight on a low-fat diet.

4. There are health consequences of a low-fat diet.

5. A low-fat diet does not promote long-term weight loss.

Let's examine each of these statements to gain some perspective on this highly controversial subject.

Americans eat too much fat   I don't have to convince anyone that Americans eat too much fat. The American palate savors the flavor of fast foods and processed foods, a change from ancestral eating habits that were rich in essential fatty acids (35 percent or more of healthy fat calories) to a diet composed of over 50 percent of calories in the form of overprocessed, health-damaging, nutrition-free, artificial fats. The health consequences of this dietary practice extend far beyond obesity into nearly every degenerative disease afflicting the human race.

It is difficult to compare a present-day diet with an ancestral diet, however, because little resemblance in the foods them-selves remains. For example, the fat content of beef eaten by an-cient peoples was about 3.9 percent. Today's beef cattle are 25 to 50 percent higher in fat, much of which is in the form of harmful arachidonic acid.[19]

An interesting book called *Native Nutrition* elaborates on the fat content of modern beef. Dr. Schmid writes:

> Tests performed by Oregon State University scientists com-pared beef from growers raising animals on mostly mother's milk and grass, with little or no grain, with USDA choice beef. Eight different cuts of each were analyzed for total fat content and for calories per pound. Naturally raised beef averaged 7.3 percent fat and 1,050 calories per pound; USDA choice beef averaged 30.0 percent fat and 1,674 calories per pound. . . . The grass-fed animals were partic-ularly lean because they were not grain fattened and be-cause they were slaughtered at ten months of age, rather than the usual eighteen. . . . The fat content of the grass-fed animals above is nearly as low as that of African grazing an-imals. . . . Generally, the fattier the beef, the more tender, tasty, and expensive it is and the more grains the animal has been fed.[20]

Betty experienced the results of a high arachidonic acid diet. Betty's country of origin, Argentina, is one of the richest cattle-producing countries in the world. Argentineans eat beef at least twice a day—fried, smothered in gravy, or worse. When Betty came to this country and started eating American-raised beef, her joints erupted in painful gout and arthritis that was only re-lieved after eliminating beef from her diet.

Contrary to what we've been told, beef is not necessarily a "bad" or fattening food, but there is some indication that the same hormones that fatten beef cattle fatten the person who eats the beef. If you're going to eat beef occasionally, you'll want to purchase natural grass-fed, organic beef from your organic grocer.

fat in the fast lane

Ever wonder about the fat content of your favorite fast food? It's not the healthy kind of fat that adds years to your years; it's the kind that hardens your arteries, causes heart disease, stroke, cancer, and other diseases of aging. Here is the fat content of America's favorite *fat* foods.[21] Keep in mind that you should try to keep your fat consumption below 35–40 grams per day.

Pizza Hut Personal Pan Pizza: 29 gr.

Taco Bell Bellgrande Nachos: 35.3 gr.

Taco Bell Taco (light): 28.8 gr.

McDonald's Big Mac: 32.4 gr.

McDonald's Chef Salad: 13.1 gr.

McDonald's Medium French Fries: 17.1 gr.

Kentucky Fried Chicken Extra Crispy Thigh: 26.3 gr.

Kentucky Fried Chicken Extra Crispy Breast: 23.7 gr.

Kentucky Fried Chicken Buttermilk Biscuit: 11.7 gr.

Burger King Scrambled Egg Platter with Sausage: 52 gr.

Burger King Bacon Double Cheeseburger Deluxe: 39 gr.

Potato chips: (1-oz. serving)

Lay's: 10 gr.

Pringle's: 13 gr.

Ruffles: 10 gr.

Wise New York Deli: 11 gr.

Pringle's Sour Cream and Onion: 12 gr.

Americans eat the wrong kinds of fat Another glimpse into ancestral diets reveals the health-conferring benefits of abundant, natural fats obtained from fish and other naturally raised animals and vegetables. Nature teaches us how valuable fats are by distributing fats bountifully throughout the food chain. Nearly every food—including fruits, vegetables, and grains—contains some form of fat. Sea foods are particularly good sources of the kinds of the omega 3 fats that reduce serum cholesterol, reduce inflammations, boost energy levels, soften the skin, nails, and hair, and confer other benefits to the body. These types of oils are simply not found in plant-based foods to the same degree.

When these naturally occurring fats are processed by heating them at extremely high temperatures, when they are heated over and over again or otherwise artificially manipulated, they are transformed from healthy fats that add life and health to our bodies into unhealthy fats that add pounds to our waistlines and subtract years from our lives.

Follow this simple rule for fat consumption: *Never, ever* eat hydrogenated fats or rancid, overheated fats. This one rule alone is worth the price of this book hundreds of times over. Hydrogenated fats from margarine and shortening, rancid fats from potato or corn chips, bacon, ham, sausages, and aged meats are toxic! Overheated fats in which French fries and other fried foods are cooked in fast-food restaurants are the *most dangerous foods* you can put into your mouth. Start working them out of your life!

Americans lose weight on a low-fat diet Nathan Pritikin proved this. Not only did his extremely low-fat, low-protein diet lower serum cholesterol and triglycerides and reduce symptoms and signs of heart disease, but excess weight dropped off as well. There were several dietary factors at work here, making it difficult to pinpoint just which dietary change or combination of changes did the work.

For the most part, people who enrolled in Pritikin's program were extremely unhealthy people. Many had already been diagnosed with heart disease and other conditions and desperately needed to make dietary changes. Not only did they restrict fat, they restricted all foods in which fat could be found and replaced them with lots of vegetables, an excellent dietary choice under any circumstances.

> *"I need to get my kids healthier. I'm setting them up. It doesn't help when Dad comes home with three bags of potato chips and a huge thing of pop."*
> **KELLY**

They also ate fruits and whole grains rich in fiber, vitamins, and minerals. Raw vegetables and fruits contain valuable enzymes that assist in the digestion and absorption of nutrients. The fiber content of the diet of those following the Pritikin plan increased dramatically, improving colon health; helping to reduce serum fats and elevated estrogens and other hormones; and in general, improving the health of the whole body.

Over time, however, the benefits from the Pritikin diet began to diminish. While the participants' hearts and arteries were healthier, they found they could not get past a certain point in their health. Something was missing from the diet, and that "something" was essential fatty acids and balanced amounts of protein.

Ann Louise Gittleman spent a number of years on the staff of the Pritikin Longevity Center as the Director of Nutrition and worked firsthand with Pritikin's diet, which allowed no more that 20 percent of caloric intake as fat. Here is what she writes about the experience:

> At the Pritikin Center where I was Director of Nutrition, I witnessed dramatic improvements in many participants who followed Pritikin's diet and whose case histories later became the statistics supporting the Pritikin program. Every day I scanned medical charts and reviewed blood values that demonstrated Pritikin's claim that "cholesterol was lowered on the average of a full 24 percent, and over 50 percent of the adult-onset diabetics leave virtually free of insulin, and after two weeks most hypertensives leave drug-free with lowered blood pressure."
>
> Shortly, however, I began to experience the downside of the Pritikin experience. Even though the participants at the Center demonstrated many positive changes while staying there, some complained of problems after leaving or when they returned for refresher courses. There were complaints about weight gain, feeling hungry all the time no matter how much food they ate, and problems because of the inordinate amount of time needed to prepare and eat six to eight small meals a day. I also noticed a rather curious phenomenon among those participants who were on the program from one to two years—the appearance of vertical ridges on the fingernails, a syndrome that signals a nutritional deficiency.[22]

Gittleman started advocating the prudent use of *added* fats and found that many of these problems were resolved immediately, *especially the unwanted weight gain!*

On the subject of Pritikin's program, Dr. Schmid writes:

That Pritikin's program has been of benefit to many individuals is undeniable. But the same program helping initially may not maintain an individual's health. Changes
away from the modern routine leading to chronic illness
(that is, changes away from sugar, refined flour, alcohol,
fatty meats, commercial dairy products, smoking, and little
or no exercise) and toward natural foods and regular exercise bring improvement and feelings of well-being.

But building lasting health and resistance to degenerative processes is more complex; there is danger in oversim-
plification. The magnitude of what has been fragmented
and mostly lost—the wisdom of our ancestors—is such that
only by being open to learning from all available sources
can one hope to put the pieces back together.[23]

Don't be fooled; the body always seeks balance. If you want
to optimize your health and maintain it for the rest of your life,
you have to balance your diet with the right amounts of carbohydrates, fats, and proteins.

There are health consequences of a low-fat diet The
health consequences of a diet too low in fat can be serious. Udo
Erasmus, author of ***Fats and Oils,*** writes:

Both LA [Linoleic Acid] and LNA [Linolenic Acid] are essential fatty acids. This means that the human body has to
have them, cannot make them, and must therefore get them
from food sources. . . . The symptoms of LA deficiency include: eczema-like skin eruptions, loss of hair, liver degeneration, behavioral disturbances, kidney degeneration,
excessive water loss through the skin accompanied by
thirst, drying up of glands, susceptibility to infections, failure of wound healing, sterility in males, miscarriage in
females, arthritis, heart and circulatory problems, and re-

tardation of growth. Prolonged absence of LA from the diet is fatal.

The symptoms of LNA deficiency include: retardation of growth, weakness, impairment of vision and learning ability, motor incoordination, tingling in arms and legs, and behavioral changes. These symptoms can be removed by adding LNA back to the diet from which it was missing. Experts have recently begun to suggest that essential fatty acid deficiency is far more widespread than was formerly believed.[24]

My clinical introduction to the dangers of a low-fat diet came when a client complained of hair loss and low levels of energy. When I asked her about her diet, she explained that she was in the process of losing weight through a prominent national weight-loss clinic. There are hundreds of these clinics throughout the country, all singing the same low-fat, low-calorie song. What she was eating was an extremely low-fat diet.

A few days later, I received a call from another woman who shared the same basic story, only worse. Her physician had put her on a *no*-fat diet.

These two women had been convinced by "the professionals" that the lower the fat content, the better the diet. Now they were suffering the consequences of this dietary foolishness. The reality is that if you want to be healthy and lose weight at the same time, you need fat. Good fat, yes. But by all means, don't try to take every gram of fat out of your diet. Not only will you stop losing weight, you'll feel terrible in the process. And just remember, one of the "side effects" of a severe deficiency in linoleic acid (one of the most *essential* of the essential fatty acids) is death.

A low-fat diet does not promote long-term weight loss
Weight loss eventually ceases on the low-fat diet. Because fat contains nine calories per gram as opposed to the four calories

per gram of both protein and carbohydrate, it seems logical to reduce calories by reducing fat. After all, if you have to reduce the weight of your wallet, take out the coins first! As one of my colleagues enjoys saying, "No matter how complex the subject of nutrition, it is never quite that simple."

To understand the mechanism of why this occurs, we must understand some of the nutritional benefits of both dietary and stored body fat—and there are many.

After water, fat is one of the most abundant substances in living beings. For example, the so-called average five-foot-four-inch woman weighing 125 pounds has, at 27 percent body fat, about 33.8 pounds of total fat, divided into 18.8 pounds of storage fat and 15 pounds of essential fats. She also has about 45 pounds of muscle, 15 pounds of bone, and 32.2 pounds of other tissue, such as blood and visceral organs.

The profile of the average man is a little different. At five feet eight inches and 154 pounds, the average man contains, at 15 percent body fat, about 23.1 pounds of fat, divided into 18.5 pounds of storage fat and 4.6 pounds of essential fat. He also has about 69 pounds of muscle, 23 pounds of bones, and 38.9 pounds of other tissue such as blood and visceral organs.[25] Don't think that storage fat is superfluous! It pads your essential organs against injury, conserves heat, and provides other benefits to the body. You don't want to lose it.

Just looking at where this fat is deposited in the body provides valuable information about its importance. Robert Erdmann, Ph.D., writes:

> The greater the chemical sensitivity of the cell, the higher the ratio will be in phosphatide's [a type of lipid or fat] favor. In vital organs or glands, such as brain, eyeball, adrenals, and testes, phosphatide levels are very high. For example, while red blood cells contain 45 percent phos-

phatide to 55 percent protein, the membranes of nerve cells contain 80 percent to 90 percent, respectively.

The more sensitive the cell is, the higher the concentration of phosphatides, and the essential fatty acids become progressively more unsaturated.[26]

Here are just a few of the functions that EFAs (essential fatty acids) perform:

EFAs are used to produce energy, from the cellular level up to the system level of the body.

EFAs govern growth, vitality, and an active mental state.

EFAs participate in the burning of food for the production of energy.

EFAs are involved in the transfer of oxygen from the air into the lungs and throughout the body.

EFAs hold oxygen in the cell membrane, acting as a barrier against viruses and bacteria.

EFAs form a structural part of all cell membranes and participate in the transfer of nutrients and other substances in and out of the cell.

EFAs help transmit messages between cells.

EFAs are burned in the mitochondria (the energy-producing part of the cell) for energy.

EFAs are precursors for prostaglandins, which regulate many functions all over the body (some of these prostaglandins lower blood pressure, relax coronary arteries, inhibit platelet stickiness).

EFAs are used to synthesize lipid/protein structures and steroid hormones.

Are you impressed yet? Can you see the importance of providing enough dietary fat to perform these vital functions? Can you see the dangers of a diet too low in essential fatty acids?

I know you want to get off this discussion of the importance of fat in your diet and back to the subject of weight loss. So let's ask the question. What role does fat play in weight maintenance? Erasmus writes:

> At levels above 12–15% of total calories, they [EFAs] increase the rate of metabolic reactions in the body, and the increased rate "burns" more fat into carbon dioxide, water and energy (heat), resulting in fat burn-off and loss of excess weight.[27]

In Ann Gittleman's [Pritikin staff member] experience, many women lose weight by making no dietary changes other than adding evening primrose oil to their daily supplement regimen. Other studies have shown that including an adequate amount of essential fatty acids from raw vegetable oils and some fish oils helps to maintain a healthy weight. And some of the "side effects" are the improved health of skin, hair, and nails, and a healthier heart.

Let's say it more clearly: You have to eat fat to lose fat! And fat must be at least 15 percent, and possibly more, of your total calories to achieve this fat-burning benefit. The type of fat you include in your diet is just as important as how much you include. I have found that a healthy diet will contain from 20 to 30 percent of caloric intake (or more for some people) as beneficial fats found abundantly in fruits, raw nuts and seeds, vegetables (like olive oil and avocados), and animal proteins like fish and organically raised poultry and beef. Vegetarians will have to be particularly careful to get enough omega 3 oils. The best way to accomplish this is by increasing the amount of flaxseed oil in the diet. (Flaxseed oils are readily available from your local health food store.)

Vegetable oils must be consumed raw with minimum processing [cold pressed] and must be kept refrigerated to preserve freshness. Oils are extremely volatile; that is, they oxidize (or become rancid) rapidly when exposed to oxygen and heat, so they must be treated delicately.

Salmon is a rich source of the beneficial EPA/DHA oils, as are other deep-sea fish. Enjoy them often. The secret to including fat in your diet is to choose your fats carefully.

the high protein diet

Now let's look at the opposite of both the high-carbohydrate and the low-fat diets. The definition of a high-protein diet is a diet that is limited in carbohydrates and includes protein in excess of the amount you personally require to maintain your body functions and structures. While this amount varies greatly from person to person, when I refer to a high-protein diet, I'm essentially discussing a diet that provides over 100 grams of protein per day.

Dr. Atkins and other authors were famous for the high-protein diets, but Atkins may have been blamed unfairly for imposing a dangerous diet on his patients. After all, his clinical records show reduction in serum fats and other health benefits, and his advice was to eat only the amount of protein a person needed—not an excessive amount.

A true high-protein, low-carbohydrate diet (the consumption of far more protein than the body requires and can use) is dangerous and will not achieve long-term weight maintenance. First, it's difficult for the kidneys to process excessive amounts of protein. Second, the weight you do lose will not be fat loss but will be primarily muscle and water weight. While Dr. Barry Sears, author of *The Zone,* has been erroneously accused of favoring high-protein diets, this is what he actually thinks of them:

These high-protein, quick-weight-loss programs have you losing the wrong kind of weight. And that's not even the worst of it. If you eat too much protein at a meal, your insulin levels will also start to increase because your body doesn't want a lot of excess amino acids floating around in the bloodstream. What will the increased insulin levels do? They now help convert the excess protein into fat.

. . . It's also been discovered recently that high-protein, ketogenic diets may cause changes in the fat cells, making them ten times more active in sequestering fat than they were before you went on the diet. So when you go off the diet, you continue to accumulate fat at a frightening rate. . . . When it [the body] has to deal with a high-protein, low-carbohydrate diet, it says, "Hey, I didn't fall off the turnip truck. The brain needs carbohydrate to function, so I'll start ripping down muscle mass, and I'll turn much of the protein in that muscle mass into carbohydrate." You might say, "That's fine. I can live with losing some muscle until I lose my body fat." But remember: Because of those increased insulin levels, you're not losing fat at anywhere near the rate you expect, and you eventually reach a weight plateau.

. . . Put this all together, and you'll see why more than 95 percent of the people who have ever lost weight using high-protein, ketogenic diets have gained that weight back and more. Why? Is everyone who ever tried a quick-weight-loss program a weak-willed ninny? I don't think so. It's just that their high-protein, low-carbohydrate diets have caused permanent changes in their fat cells, changes that virtually guarantee increased body-fat accumulation in the future.[28]

An eating plan that balances protein, carbohydrates, and fats is the only one that will work toward permanent, healthy weight maintenance. Before we discuss that plan in more detail, let's look at the siren call of the dieting world: herbal weight-loss products.

the herbal weight-loss diet

Regardless of how eloquently and passionately we state our position that you must change how you eat if you want to lose weight and keep it off, I know there's a segment of the population that wants to skip through every chapter that covers dietary restrictions and go directly to the words "If you take this pill, you can lose weight without making any sacrifices at all." If that's the level of your commitment, you may as well stop reading this book right now.

Weight-loss pills are marketed so aggressively through health food stores, multilevel companies (your next-door neighbor or sister-in-law, for example), drugstores, TV commercials, and mail-order catalogs that it's tempting to believe the hype. Maybe it's true that pills can dissolve fat off your waist as efficiently as Liquid-Plumr dissolves the sludge in your bathroom drain.

Over the past few months I've seen literally hundreds of signs decorating the roadways, promising to help me lose fifteen pounds in fifteen days, thirty pounds in thirty days, guaranteed weight loss or my money back. They promise to increase my energy while the weight just drops off.

Some of these signs are hand-lettered on brown cardboard

box lids; some are run off a copier at a local print shop. Most are tacked onto telephone poles or on stakes stuck into the ground at busy intersections. It always seems a little odd that *someone, somewhere* actually expects people to write down the phone number off a fence post and call someone they have never met, buy a product about which they know nothing—from a company that may or may not be ethical or competent, and put that product into their bodies! It's even odder that many people actually do this!

I've investigated scores of these products and found them *without exception* to be products of inferior quality, sold at exorbitant prices, and predicated on pseudoscience that will render the user worse off than when he or she started using the product.

What the advertisements don't say is that while I'm speedily dropping the weight, I'm losing valuable cellular water stores and depleting the energy of some of the most critical organs in my body. In other words, while I'm losing pounds, I'm losing my health.

How Do Herbal Weight-Loss Products Work?

The most popular herbal products on the market contain a veritable bouquet of some of the most stimulating herbs on earth, like guarana, ephedra (or ma huang), kola or bissey nut, capsicum or cayenne pepper, and others. While small amounts of these herbs have benefits that do not include weight loss, they were never intended to be combined to stimulate the body so violently.

Symptoms that accompany the use of these products can include nervousness, agitation, hand tremor, insomnia, palpitations, trembling, weakness, sweating, a feeling of warmth, chilly sensation, nausea, and vomiting. Other side effects include nervousness, headache, insomnia, dyspnea or shortness of breath, a tired feeling, thirst, drowsiness, feeling of distress in the area of the heart and stomach, flushing of the skin, tingling and numbness of the extremities, anorexia, constipation, quivering feeling, faintness and diuresis (excessive urination).[29] Users of excessive amounts of herbal stimulants may experience elevated blood pressure.

Yes, these herbal combinations may make a person feel a surge in energy. It feels good after the exhaustion caused by low thyroid function, poor dietary choices, insufficient adrenal output, or possibly hundreds of other conditions that have left the person feeling exhausted. Unfortunately, the type of energy users now feel is what we nutritionists call a "false high." The energy they are experiencing is not the type of sustained energy that comes from improving the health of the body or from providing superior nutrition to feed the energy-hungry cells of the body. It comes rather at the expense of the endocrine system by over-stimulating the adrenals and sending the central nervous system into a frenzy of activity.

Many users of herbal weight-loss products describe the feeling they get from ephedra-based products as the same type of high they experienced using recreational drugs. And many of them have become just as addicted to herbal stimulants as they were to street drugs.

> *"I don't know why I'm eating this . . . but I can't help it! I was just craving . . . I just wanted to eat it, so I did. I was possessed."*
> **JANE**

One client recently discussed her personal history of drug use that dates back a couple of decades into her teens and twenties when she used a substantial amount of uppers and other drugs. When she got married, she abandoned her drug habit and gave birth to several children. With the birth of each child, her energy levels dropped lower and lower until finally, after the last child was born, she hardly had the strength to pull herself off the couch and take care of them. Obviously, the nutritional needs of her body had not been met during her childbearing years!

Finally, in an attempt to get her health and energy back, she enrolled in an aerobics class at a local gym with a group of other young mothers. One day while discussing her declining energy levels, one of the moms pulled her aside and said, "You know, I used to feel the same way, but now I use herbal weight-loss products that contain ephedra, and my old energy is back. Don't worry; they are totally natural so they are safe. You can buy them at your local health food store . . ."

Our young mother visited her health food store. Sure enough, she saw a stack of herbal weight-loss pills displayed prominently on the counter, laced with enough ephedra to pull up her energy and pull down her adrenal gland. She bought a bottle and started taking them. Before long, her energy was up to what she remembered it could be but she described the experience this way: "It feels like I'm back on street drugs. Can this be good for me?"

She had reason to be concerned. If she continued to use the products, her critical energy shortage would drop even further. Sooner or later, she would face the consequences in a burned-out adrenal gland and an exhausted nervous system. I worked with her over several months to wean her off the herbal products, then put her on nutrients to restore her own natural energy. It may take her a year or more to recuperate!

AN HERBAL A DAY

Some herbal products work by increasing the elimination of water with diuretics or stimulating bowel function by laxatives. These products typically use such herbs as corn silk, uva ursi, cascara sagrada, senna, and others.

Several years ago I tested both body fat and body water levels of several dozen dieters. The important water supply was deficient by at least 1 percent in every person who had been using herbal diuretics. Some were deficient by several percent. This may not seem significant until you realize that by the time you are thirsty, you are already 1 percent dehydrated; 5 percent dehydration can lead to serious health problems, and 10 percent dehydration is death! Every percent of water content of the body is critical!

Continued use of laxative herbs like cascara sagrada and senna is addictive. Over time, the ability to maintain normal bowel function without the herbs is lost. And really, what's the point of weight loss? Is it just a few pounds on the scale, or is it *fat* loss?

No herbal diuretic or laxative can help you lose fat tissue. Any advertisement that promises to help you lose so much weight in so many days is promising water loss, not fat loss. It is biochemically impossible to lose *fat* that quickly! What you really need to do is balance your body; i.e., bring your body into homeostatic balance so that the excess *fat* drops off as a consequence of balanced nutrition. That is the only guaranteed *safe* way to do it.

The moral of the story is clear: Herbal weight-loss products are not safe. While they promise instant results, they can't fulfill their promises, and you are left poorer at the end after you have used them. Don't be tempted by the hype. You're much too smart for that.

now the good news!

There is an answer to weight loss, and it is permanent—as long as you stick with the program. It isn't difficult, it won't leave you starving for a "real meal," and it doesn't involve weird foods. It's just a little different, but you can do it. Later in the book we'll look carefully at how you really can lose your weight, forever, and increase your health and vitality with every delicious bite you take. But the first step is to learn how to listen to your body.

Learn what "feels satisfied" and then eat only to the point of satisfaction. Eat just the amount of food that is right for you. Sound too simple? It may not be as simple as you think! For example, do you feel guilty if you leave food on your plate and dutifully eat it all, even if it's too much food? Stop feeling guilty! Is it morally preferable to waste food by overeating and ruining your body than to waste it by scraping it into the garbage can?

Eat slowly; when you're satisfied, stop eating! This simple rule includes guilt-induced eating, which is a little tougher to deal with. Do you live with or associate with someone who insists on feeding you food you'd rather not eat? I call these people "loving saboteurs." They think they know what is best for you and encourage you to overindulge or eat the wrong foods. I have a "loving saboteur" in my life whom I love dearly, but I've learned that when he cuts a piece of birthday cake that is twice the size I requested, I eat what I want and leave the rest on my plate. And I don't feel guilty. After all, I'm in charge of my body!

A saboteur can be that wife or mom who shows her love by baking chocolate chip cookies when you prefer fresh fruit, or fried chicken when you prefer baked. It may be that husband who surprises his dieting wife with a two-pound box of truffles for her birthday (when she requested an exercise bike!). It may be that coworker who brings a box of cream-filled donuts to the office, waves it under your nose, and mocks you when you refuse. Or the next-door neighbor who rings your doorbell and offers a fat-filled casserole as a peace offering, or your best friend who invites you for coffee and cake and insists she'll be hurt if you leave any on your plate. You simply must learn to take charge of what goes into your mouth.

Taking charge of your weight means taking charge of what you eat, and you can start that process immediately!

But now you need to understand more about how your own body may be working against you, even with the best diet in the world. We'll look at six issues that simply must be addressed if you are going to lose weight and keep it off permanently. And then we'll share some important information on how to deal with those issues. The first issue is your own body fat and how to get it working *for* you instead of *against* you!

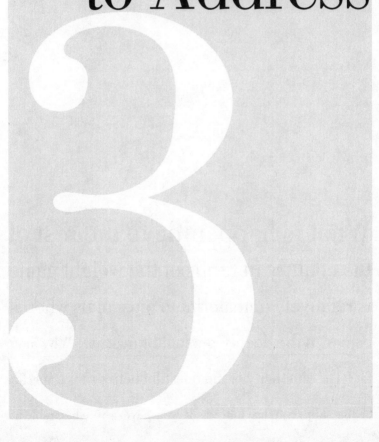

Six
Problems
You Need
to Address

3

What is happening to the rest of the country in terms of the weight game is relatively immaterial to most of us when it comes to the deeply personal question: Why am *I* fat? The simplicity of the question belies the complexity of the subject. Why, indeed, do you have a weight problem?

Are you overweight because you overeat? Are you overweight because of a thyroid imbalance? An estrogen imbalance? Did you gain your excess pounds after the birth of your children and just can't get it off? Do you crave inappropriate foods like chocolate, fat, or salt? Would you rather sponsor a bake sale than a bike ride? Do you frequently binge and purge?

Questions about the causes of obesity are many and varied because the reasons behind poor weight management are many and varied. And maybe this is the reason diets fail: Diets don't address the complexity of the problem of weight control.

Amidst all the hoopla and hurrahs of new diets and eating programs, don't forget that the maintenance of a healthy weight (and a healthy body) is a complex issue that touches on the endocrine system, the digestive system, and the elimination system. It revolves around what you eat and why you eat it, how you prepare it, and how you balance it with other nutrients. Those extra 25 or 125 pounds you carry on your hips and thighs will not come off just from wishful thinking—and certainly not by following the latest in diet fashion.

In chapter 2 we talked about the critical non-role of calorie counting and how a diet that is too low in calories sets you up for dietary failure. Now let's look at the first of six reasons why you may have been unable to lose weight on any other program. This first problem is a different aspect of calories—your body's ability (or lack thereof) to waste them.

you may have insufficient BAT

Late one summer afternoon, I received a call from our nutritional counselor at the medical clinic. "Carol, I think you need to talk with one of our patients. She's about seventy-five pounds overweight and can't lose it. We've put her on a calorie-restricted diet, on a carbohydrate-restricted diet, and on a fat-restricted diet. We've checked her thyroid and her hormones, but nothing works. She's desperate!"

Wow. I love a challenge, but I wasn't sure I wanted to undertake this one. I agreed to call her. Sure enough. She was not a happy woman. She elaborated on the counselor's story, telling me about the enormous stress she had been under the past few years, how obesity had changed her life drastically and that if she didn't lose the weight, she really didn't want to live!

When confronted with a client who doesn't do well on tested and tried protocol, it's tempting to say, "Well, obviously she's not complying with the diet." But I find that approach so demeaning, so professionally uncaring and self-serving, that I can't do it.

Here was a woman who was obviously motivated to change her diet but even with the best of intentions and strictest compliance, the scales didn't budge. The doctor and I started looking for other answers and found the solution in the unlikeliest place—her own store of body fat. What we're talking about here is two kinds of fat, both of which are beneficial in the right amounts and are involved in the burning of excess calories.

The body fat we're all familiar with is what scientists call White Adipose Tissue (WAT). WAT helps to insulate our internal organs from the cold and cushions them from shock and trauma. It acts as a storage depot for toxic materials that burden the liver, and it serves as an emergency source of energy when the food supply runs low. However, WAT is metabolically inert. That is, it's incapable of contributing much energy or heat to the body.

The primary job of every cell in the body is the production of energy which keeps the body alive and functional. Carbohydrates, fats, and to a lesser degree proteins are drawn into the cell and through a complicated series of biochemical events, are burned to produce heat and energy, much the same way that wood or oil stoked into a furnace provides heat for our homes and offices.

> *"At forty-three, I'm just coming into my prime. I want to get better, feel better, so I'm not embarrassed to put on a pair of shorts, take off with my kids, and do things with them."*
> **JANE**

Think of each cell as a tiny energy-burning factory. These little factories contain mitochondria, the site of energy production. Some cells contain only a few mitochondria; others contain hundreds or thousands. Tissues that are metabolically very active, as is liver tissue, contain up to 2,000 mitochondria per cell. A human egg (the ovum) may contain up to 300,000 mitochondria per cell. (Never underestimate the power of a woman!) WAT cells, on the other hand, contain only one or two mitochondria; over 85 percent of the total WAT cell volume is a globule of fat.

However, there is a metabolically active form of body fat, not so well known, whose importance is just now becoming a hot research topic in some major research institutions around the world. Brown fat, or Brown Adipose Tissue (BAT), stimulates thermogenesis or the production of heat. If researchers can discover how to use this type of fat more efficiently, they just might reduce the world's weight problem once and for all.

BAT is formed in utero at about the twentieth week and is deposited primarily in the back of the neck, throughout the organs in the abdomen, between the shoulder blades, around the blood vessels in the thoracic region (the heart and lungs), on top of the kidneys, beside the breast bone, beside large blood vessels, and especially along the spinal cord and key bones. The position of BAT throughout the body keeps key organs warm and disperses heat throughout the rest of the body.

For a period of several months or years after a child is born, BAT actively burns calories to produce heat through a process called Cold Induced Non-Shivering Thermogenesis (CINST). Ever notice that babies never shiver? They don't need to. BAT keeps them warm, much in the same way that bears and other hibernating animals sleep through the cold winter months without suffering from hypothermia.

BAT is not the only organ in the body that produces heat, which we will see in the next chapter on the thyroid gland. Certain organs of the endocrine system maintain their own thermostat, which can lower or raise the core temperature as needed to keep the body at 98.6 degrees. However, if BAT is present in sufficient quantities or *is actively functioning*, our bodies will be much more efficient, not only in the production of heat but also in burning excess calories.

It is in the burning of heat through the wasting of calories that we begin to see the value of BAT from the standpoint of the dieter. As we discussed in chapter 2, associating calorie counting with weight control becomes a meaningless exercise because calorie requirements fluctuate from day to day, from moment to moment, depending on both internal and external conditions.

If your body is not efficient at wasting unneeded calories via BAT activation, you can't help but gain weight, *regardless of how few calories you consume!* The very process of food restriction can cause the thermogenic process to shut down because the body becomes more efficient. As we reduce food consumption, we don't need as much energy to fuel the body, and it slows down further and further. Finally the body begins to store calories instead of wasting them.

WHEN YOUR BODY CAN'T "WASTE" CALORIES

Let's tie these two subjects together. We have seen that embarking on a low-calorie diet sets in motion a chain of metabolic events, the culmination of which is a shutdown of the basal metabolic rate (BMR). As calories diminish, so does the body's ability to use them. According to some researchers, regardless of how few calories we consume, there is an inevitable 15 percent "waste factor" built in, that only about 85 percent of all ingested calories are used to meet basic energy demands or the energy required to keep the body alive and functioning. The other 15 percent of ingested calories must be dealt with.

Until recently, scientists thought the body had only one way to deal with excess calories—storage—and so fat-reducing programs were centered on just one concept: calorie restriction. It has been only in the last few years that scientists have begun to realize the importance of BAT in dealing with those excess calories in a more constructive way than simply storing them on the hips.

For normal-weight people, BAT works to eliminate the negative impact of excess calories by burning or "wasting" them in the production of body heat. Individuals who struggle with chronic weight challenges, however, may have lost the assistance of brown fat. For them, the body really does have no choice other than to store those 15 percent excess calories. For some people, especially those who cycle weight loss, their bodies have become calorie misers—energy scrooges that desperately hang on to every calorie, packing it away into storage for another day.

> *"I don't feel comfortable
> running across the baseball
> field with my girls; I feel like
> Jurassic Park."*
> **JANE**

Genetics may also be a dominant force in the function of brown fat. Some individuals may simply be born with either inadequate amounts of BAT or their own stores of BAT are depleted for other reasons, including excessive exercise, fasting, breast-feeding, diabetes, dressing too warmly, pregnancy, fever, and hypothalamic lesions.[1]

For others of us, the aging process or obesity begins to take its toll, and the mitochondria in brown fat begins to shut down. Reduced BAT activity can also reduce thyroid function. As the thyroid gland slows down its activity and lowers body temperature even further, a layer of white fat builds up around the internal organs, further insulating them against lower temperatures and further reducing the need for brown fat to produce heat. The downward cycle spirals faster and faster. In the process BAT is turned into WAT, becoming metabolically inactive by losing the activity of the mitochondria and shutting down the ability of the body to create heat and waste calories.

This is when, for many people, losing weight becomes an impossible dream. It simply doesn't happen, no matter how good the diet or how compliant the dieter.

INCREASING YOUR BAT-TING AVERAGE

You can restimulate BAT by a variety of means. One way is through eating foods rich in essential fats, particularly GLA (gamma linoleic acid) from the evening primrose or borage oils, or foods containing a rich supply of carnitine (animal proteins).

Some research has been done on the effect of cold temperatures on BAT. The theory is that exposing an individual to a cold environment for long periods of time will eventually kick in the thermogenic propensity of the body in self-defense. The problem is, not many people are willing to strip down to their underwear in a refrigeration unit for weeks at a time just to lose weight!

Several antiobesity drugs on the market today are geared toward stimulating the central nervous system (CNS) to stimulate the activity of BAT. The problem is that significant side effects, such as disturbed heart rhythms, accompany the use of these drugs.

While drug researchers are working to put together a team of pharmaceutical agents that effectively but safely stimulate brown fat, dozens of herbal companies have been working on the same thing through the use of natural stimulants like ma huang (ephedra) and caffeine-containing herbs. While these herbal combinations are marketed as totally safe—a natural alternative to drugs—the vast majority are *not* safe. A number of people have died, and others have suffered from significant side effects (including adrenal exhaustion, CNS disorders, and heart arrhythmias) as a result of using these herbs over a long period of time. (See pp. 56–60 for more information about herbal weight-loss programs.)

However, a number of researchers are hard at work on a class of herbal agents that *safely* stimulate the activity of the central nervous system and reactivate brown adipose tissue. Work is currently being done at Brigham Young University using a combination of herbs and over-the-counter drugs that causes the reactivation of BAT without the accompanying side effects that have made even herbal combinations unsafe for public use.

There are *safe* herbal products, and I learned that they can be used effectively for those clients who can't lose weight any other way. Remember the woman at the beginning of the chapter? After discussing my client's needs with her physician, I put her on a safe, well-balanced herbal formula to stimulate thermogenesis and sat back nervously to wait. If this failed, I dreaded talking with her again. After waiting in vain for six weeks for the phone to ring, I finally called her.

"I only call when I'm upset," she explained. "So far I've lost thirty-five pounds. I feel fabulous—better than I have for years—and the weight is still dropping. I'll be down to my ideal weight by Christmas. I'm following your diet recommendations, too!"

If you are interested in pursuing BAT thermogenesis and the herbal combination that has been safely used in research studies, I encourage you to contact the American Phytotherapy Research Laboratory in Utah for more information (see Appendix C). The herbal combination used in the research is available through many health food stores under the brand name Silver Sage Thermogenics Plus.

your body may be storing toxic waste

If you're overweight, chances are you're not a glutton, but you probably do eat too many nonfoods. Some nutritionists call these "food artifacts," or products made by human workmanship. These are substances that are not naturally present in the world and were not part of our ancestors' diets.

A graphic way to illustrate the cultural shift our country has experienced in terms of what we stuff into our mouths is to share some actual food diaries from two of my weight-loss clients. These lists are more "normal" than you would think.

Day 1

Breakfast: 20-oz. root beer
Lunch: bread stick, 2 candy bars, 20-oz. root beer
Dinner: hot dog with bun and corn
Snack: caramel corn

Day 2:

Breakfast: 20-oz. root beer
Lunch: 20-oz. root beer and a deli sandwich
Dinner: tomato soup with a tuna-fish sandwich
Snack: bowl of ice cream

Day 3:

Breakfast: 20-oz soft drink
Lunch: nothing
Dinner: nothing
Snack: beef jerky

Day 4

Breakfast: nothing
Lunch: bagel with cream cheese with a soft drink
Dinner: spaghetti with mushroom sauce, with soft drink
Snack: 2 20-oz. soft drinks

Day 5

Breakfast: nothing
Lunch: banana bread with carrots and soft drink
Dinner: Whopper with french fries and soft drink
Snack: caramel corn with saltwater taffy

Day 6

Breakfast: banana bread

Lunch: apple, beef jerky, and a soft drink
Dinner: chicken, potato, corn, and a soft drink
Snack: saltwater taffy

Let's analyze this six-day food diary from the perspective of a nutritionist, although one doesn't need expert advice to see what's wrong with this picture. In six days, this individual ate a total of three servings of vegetables, only one of which was fresh (the potato on Day 6). She ate only one serving of fruit, two servings of high-quality protein, and the rest was junk.

In my lectures, I often comment that people can eat three meals a day, seven days a week, and eat no food at all. The audience stares back in disbelief. How can this be true? And yet, when you look at a diary such as the one above, it's easy to see it in black and white.

Here's what another client ate for one week:

Day 1

Breakfast: one slice of sourdough bread
Lunch: bacon, lettuce, and tomato sandwich
Dinner: hot dog and 1 cup of cottage cheese
Snack: coffee with cream and chewing gum

Day 2

Breakfast: slice of toast with peanut butter and apple butter
Lunch: 1 cup of highly sweetened yogurt with banana bread
Dinner: frozen tuna noodle casserole

Day 3

Breakfast: peanut butter and jam sandwich with a glass of orange juice (frozen concentrate)
Lunch: raisins
Dinner: four pieces of fried chicken

Day 4

Breakfast: peanut butter and jam sandwich
Lunch: one-quarter glass of orange juice
Dinner: nothing:
Snack: 1 cup of coffee with cream

Day 5

Breakfast: homemade chocolate chip cookies
Lunch: 1 cup of milk
Dinner: Thanksgiving dinner (the works!)
Snack: one cup of coffee with cream and some candy

Day 6

Breakfast: peanut butter and jam sandwich with chocolate chip cookies
Lunch: 1 cup of raw cabbage
Dinner: hot dog with bun
Snack: four pieces of chocolate cake, with two ounces of hard candy

Day 7

Breakfast: slice of toast with peanut butter
Lunch: banana bread
Snack: cereal with milk
Dinner: chicken and mushroom casserole
Snack: raisins

If you look at supermarket stats, you'll see what Americans are buying—and it isn't food. We're eating more pseudofood now than ever in the history of the world. And don't think your body doesn't know the difference. That entrée may taste and smell like real food, but your body knows otherwise, and it knows where to store every toxic molecule. All the low-fat this and low-fat that, the sugar substitute here and the fat substitute there will not solve your fat problem.

Over 75 percent of the food products sold in our supermarkets are either nutritionally dead or nutritionally toxic. We don't bury that dead food; we store it on our hips, waists, and chests, pound after pound after pound. Why build more toxic waste dumps in this country when we can use our bodies instead?

FAT—THE TOXIC WASTE DEPOT

Food takes a simple route in our bodies: It is chewed, swallowed, digested into its elemental parts, received into the body, and used for thousands of metabolic functions and for building such key structures as muscles, blood, and skin. Unusable metabolic by-products and waste materials are filtered through the kidneys and liver and excreted from the body. It's an efficient system that has worked well since the creation of humankind.

But what happens when modern food products that bear little resemblance to real food are chewed, swallowed, and broken down into their elemental fragments? The body now has two problems to solve: It is left without the very elements it needs to fuel the body's metabolic processes and it is encumbered with *stuff* for which it has no use.

Think of a bicycle factory that orders wheels, chains, bars, screws, and seat cushions to stock the assembly line but instead receives packing crates stuffed with Styrofoam peanuts or wood shavings. Not only does the assembly line shut down because the raw materials are not available, but the workers have to get rid of the junk that's accumulating in the back room.

What does this analogy have to do with excess body weight? Fat performs an important function in the body by storing toxic waste. We don't like to think of ourselves as carrying around a load of biochemical poisons, but the fact is, we're not able to ex-

crete all the endogenous (created by bodily processes) and ex-
ogenous (ingested from the outside) poisons to which we're exposed.

It's the kidney's and the liver's job to remove waste material
from the body. When we eat foods our bodies can't use, or foods
that contain artificial ingredients; when we breathe polluted air;
when our digestive systems do not sufficiently break down the
foods into usable parts, the liver is required to handle an excessive amount of toxic waste for which it is not prepared.

Most of us don't drink enough water or eat enough fiber for
the colon and kidneys to perform their vital functions, and waste
materials build up in the colon to be reabsorbed into the body.

Symptoms of inadequate waste disposal may include constipation (less than one to two easy bowel movements per day), bad
breath, low energy, bloated abdomen, coated tongue, and skin
eruptions, and may be a factor in many degenerative diseases.
Constipation is an extremely common health problem. Many
doctors disagree with our definition of constipation and tell patients that "normal" bowel evacuation can range from once or
twice each day to once or twice each week.

> *"You feel so good when
> you're eating that chocolate
> cake or that ice cream, but
> then after you feel so bad.
> That's part of the addiction."*
> **MONTE**

Imagine sitting down to enjoy a meal and chewing each little
bite, then spitting the food into an enamel pan instead of swal-

lowing. After the meal, you place the pan in an oven at a temperature of about 98.6 degrees. You do this at breakfast, lunch, and dinner, and one or two snacks throughout the day. You let the pan sit in the oven for one day, then two days, then three days . . . or however long is "normal" for you. Imagine the foul odor that would soon permeate your house.

Now replace the enamel pan in the oven with your colon and intestines. Unless you move your bowels every day at least once, and preferably twice, fecal material is rotting and fermenting in that warm, moist environment! Fortunately, you can't smell it (unless you have body odor or bad breath), but the damage it does to your body is incalculable. Frequent, regular bowel movements are a critical part of nurturing a healthy body and will help keep your weight in check as well.

Logic tells us that if we clean up our diets and eat pure foods, including thirty to forty grams of fiber a day, drink eight to ten glasses of water, and avoid synthetic chemicals as much as possible, our bodies will not have to build storage depots on our hips and bellies to handle an unnecessary load of toxic waste. While a moderate amount of stored fat protects the heart, kidneys, and other internal organs from shock, provides a rich source of energy, insulates the body against sudden changes in temperature, cushions the posterior when sitting for long periods of time, and in general, makes the body more attractive, fat should not be considered a dumping ground for the metabolic by-products of junk food. But that is, in fact, what excess body fat can be.

By the way, weight loss should be gradual. When you lose fat, the toxic materials stored in the tissue can be released into the bloodstream on their way out of the body. The release of too many toxins too quickly into the bloodstream can place undue stress on the body. One to two pounds of fat loss per week is just about perfect for everyone.

you may be allergic to your favorite foods

Allergies are an extremely common cause of weight gain. Since virtually everyone is allergic to something, even if they don't recognize the symptoms, we need to explore in more depth the topic of allergies as they relate to excessive weight.

Nadine loves bread. She loves pasta and sweet rolls. She loves anything with wheat in it, and because she works in a coffee shop that sells the most delectable rolls and cookies hot from the oven, she has indulged freely. But when she went on our eating program, which effectively eliminates *all* wheat products, she found the weight dropping off. Part of her weight loss was the new balance in food, but part of it could have been that she was no longer consuming this highly allergic food which her body stored on her hips.

She had a chance to test her allergy a few weeks later. One afternoon her husband graciously served fresh turkey sandwiches. He used only the finest whole-grain, high-fiber bread, piled it high with roasted turkey, lettuce, and slices of tomato, moistened it with a little mayonnaise, and Nadine enjoyed every delicious morsel.

Within minutes of swallowing the last crumb, she got so sleepy she couldn't hold her eyes open, and she lay down to take a little nap. She said she felt like she was in a coma.

Turkey is high in tryptophan, which can produce a sedative effect. (Remember how you feel shortly after Thanksgiving dinner!) When I asked Nadine if turkey ever did that to her, she replied, "No, we have turkey all the time. The only thing I hadn't eaten for a while was the bread. It had to be the bread." She recalled that before she went on the diet, she tended to get sleepy after eating wheat products but had never associated the two events.

Nadine's story is not uncommon. Wheat often causes symptoms such as depression, inappropriate sleepiness, headaches, gastrointestinal upsets, arthritic pains, and almost any other symptom imaginable in any part of the body.

Wheat isn't the only bad guy here. Let me share some really bad news with you: The food you crave desperately or the food you love the most is typically the food to which you are allergic. Almost every time.

We've all heard the expression: "One man's food is another man's poison." We're not talking here about eating synthetic foodlike products that have no biological activity in the human body. We're not talking about food additives, preservatives, coloring agents, flavor enhancers, or the like, although these agents may certainly produce the same effects. We are talking about *good* foods that nourish other people: foods like milk, yogurt, cheese, corn, soy, chocolate.

The real question is why do we become allergic or reactive to common foods that don't affect other people? There are several causes of allergy, not the least of which is genetics. We can inherit allergic tendencies from ancestors, even though we may not be allergic to the same foods. Allergies have been a real issue in several generations of both my husband's family and mine, so when our children tested high for food sensitivities, we weren't surprised.

A theory that is difficult to prove but interesting to contemplate is that our bodies have difficulty distinguishing between chemicals secreted by negative emotions and the foods we happen to be eating when we experience these emotions. One reason we shouldn't eat when we're upset is that negative emotions can shut down the digestive system, which can cause undigested proteins to be received into the body and attacked by an overzealous immune system. If we're eating a peanut butter and jelly sandwich while we're being disciplined for sloppy table manners or get angry when being kicked under the table by an older brother, our bodies may associate that peanut butter sandwich with depression, frustration, or anger and initiate an allergic response upon every exposure to peanuts, bread, or jelly!

> *"My dad would always harass my mom about her weight and she would ignore him or get mad at him. It was okay for him to be overweight but not for my mom. Men think that a man can be heavy and it's perfect."*
>
> **BETH**

If we consoled ourselves during a time of grief or depression with Oreo cookies and a glass of milk, possibly any exposure to chocolate or milk reproduces the same feelings of depression or grief. Or if we just happened to eat a piece of toast while suffering from a raging headache, the body now connects the headache and the toast—and reproduces the effect year after year.

A number of years ago, I experienced a devastating bout of stomach flu that lasted for weeks. The last food item I ate before I started vomiting was a certain brand of shortbread cookies. For years after recovering from the flu, my stomach lurched every time I passed a package of shortbread cookies in the cookie aisle of the supermarket. Maybe we develop our own unique set of allergens the same way. Our bodies just can't separate those events from the internal chemicals they produce.

Strong adrenal glands help protect us from the negative side effects of stress. If the adrenal glands have been weakened by unrelenting stress, drugs, or illness, we may become increasingly reactive to foods and other environmental chemicals.

Other adrenal-weakening factors include deficiencies in key nutrients like vitamin C and pantothenic acid; excessive consumption of coffee, alcohol, sugar, and other central nervous system stimulants or depressants; or recreational drugs. If you find that you simply can't wake up in the morning without your morning cup of coffee and sugar-coated donut, chances are good that you're self-medicating with caffeine and sugar to support a barely functional adrenal gland. You are setting yourself up for food and airborne allergies.

Another common cause of allergy is incomplete digestion. This is a complex function that frankly doesn't get done very efficiently for most of us.

The first step of digestion begins in the mouth where the teeth chew and grind the food into tiny fragments and mix it with saliva. Saliva contains small amounts of amylase, an enzyme that helps break down carbohydrates into simple sugars. When the food is swallowed, it rests in the upper portion of the stomach (the cardiac region) for up to an hour. If the food was raw and contained its own supply of enzymes, the warmth and moisture of the stomach allow the enzymes in the raw food to take the next step in the process of digestion and break it down further.

The food remains in the cardiac region of the stomach for about thirty to forty minutes, during which time the lower portion of the stomach (the duodenal portion) prepares to receive the partially digested food by secreting its own digestive juices, including pepsin and hydrochloric acid (HCL). The HCL turns the pepsin into pepsinogen, which then cleaves the protein molecules into individual amino acids. After passing from the stomach into the small intestine in the form of chyme, the food continues to be further digested and absorbed all along the digestive tract.

> *"You go to the store, kids*
> *make comments. It makes*
> *you feel real conscious when*
> *you're buying things. People*
> *look at you like they're*
> *saying, 'Wow, she really*
> *needs that!'"*
> **CASSIE**

Each section of the digestive tract contains juices that break down the food into smaller and smaller particles, each step critical in the overall digestive process. Protein digestion takes place primarily in the stomach and small intestine. Carbohydrate digestion takes place in the mouth, stomach, and small intestine. Fat digestion takes place in the small intestine. Conditions along the entire length of the alimentary canal must be optimum for full digestion to take place, and it doesn't take much imagination to realize that with most people, optimum conditions rarely exist.

When digestion is incomplete, particles of undigested food pass through the small intestine. Constipation, harmful bacterium and yeasts, and malnutrition can riddle the walls of the small intestine with tiny holes that allow entry of these large, undigested protein and carbohydrate particles directly into the bloodstream. At this point the immune system becomes involved.

The job of the immune system is to recognize and destroy foreign invaders, proteins, or other objects that don't belong in the bloodstream. When an immune body homes in on a partially digested protein molecule, it calls out the body's armed forces. It matters little to the immune body that the protein molecule on which it has sent out a "search and destroy" mission is an innocuous glass of milk or a slice of toast with peanut butter. It may not know that most of the world has no problem with walnuts; it only knows that this tiny cluster of amino acids doesn't match up to "self"; it must be destroyed.

It doesn't seem practical to call out the armed forces when one foreign soldier steps foot over the border, but that is essentially what the body does when undigested food slips through the intestinal barrier into the bloodstream. Although everyone else may enjoy a piece of whole wheat toast with peanut butter and jam, your body may not perceive that piece of toast as food. It may set out to eliminate it from the body in a variety of interesting ways, including diarrhea; sneezing; itchy, watery eyes; headaches; or vomiting. It can "seal off" toxins by chronic constipation or encasing them in adipose tissue; i.e., fat cells. If the body has to deal with large amounts of these toxic by-products of poor digestion or allergies, it may need to build large storage depots of fat all over the body to handle the load.

Another common technique the body uses to deal with allergic material is to flood the affected area with water, a condition we recognize as water retention or edema. People can lose ten to twenty pounds of excess fluid just by eliminating allergic foods from their diet.

TROUBLESOME FOODS

The most allergenic foods in the American diet are the foods we consume the most frequently, namely corn, wheat, dairy products, peanuts, citrus, soy, eggs, and to a lesser degree, nuts. Sugar is another common allergen, although sugar is harmful in other ways as well.

People often become allergic to food just because they eat the same foods too frequently. We eat virtually the same twenty foods every day of our lives! As a nutritionist, I study the dietary patterns of my clients and see what they eat on a day-to-day basis. A typical "healthy" American menu looks like this:

Breakfast:

Slice of whole-grain toast with butter or margarine and jam
Cup of coffee with sugar and cream
Bowl of whole-grain cereal with milk
Glass of reconstituted orange juice sweetened with fructose or corn syrup

Lunch:

Sandwich with processed meat or a fast-food hamburger

Dinner:

Pasta with tomato or butter sauce (or a protein-based entrée)
Salad (iceberg lettuce and highly processed dressing)
French bread with a little butter
Dessert, often with coffee and sugar

Do you see the common thread of wheat, corn, dairy, and sugar running through this typical American menu? Not only is this type of diet deficient in a number of critical nutrients, including protein and fats, it is also a highly pro-allergenic diet.

If you're going to get your allergies under control and thus help bring your weight into line, look closely at your current diet. What foods do you love the most? What foods can you absolutely *not* live without? What foods do you eat every day? These may be the foods to which you are allergic and should consider eliminating from your diet for at least six weeks. You may drop ten to fifteen pounds just from this simple effort.

The recipes and menus outlined in chapter 8 and Appendix A are designed to avoid most common allergens. Now is an excellent time to start ridding your diet of your allergenic foods. If you follow my food plan very carefully for several weeks, and then eat a food to which you are allergic after having avoided it during that time, you will usually experience a marked response to that food—an increased allergic reaction. To explain this heightened response, imagine a man who is sleeping on a bed of nails. If you remove one of those nails, he won't notice. But let him sleep on a feather bed for a few nights, and then introduce just one nail into the mattress; he will notice it immediately!

Think of your food allergies as nails. Your body is struggling to adapt to the presence of those allergens and often will develop an addiction to that food as part of its adaptive process. If you remove all the allergens, let your body calm down and establish harmony, and then invite the offending substance back in, your body will protest immediately.

Typical allergic symptoms can include digestive upsets (bloating, belching, diarrhea, constipation, alternating diarrhea/constipation), skin eruptions, headaches, depression, sinus infections, frequent bronchial inflammations, fleeting aches and pains, arthritis, palpitations of the heart, inappropriate sleepiness, and of course, weight gain, and many others.

Learn to "read" your body. Dairy products frequently cause sinus infections or oozing sinuses (mucous dripping down the back of the throat) and diarrhea or constipation. Typical symptoms of wheat allergy include headaches, depression, midafternoon sleepiness, snoring, and other mental disorders. But again, any food can cause literally any reaction. Be on the alert for allergies.

you may be gaining weight from prescription drugs

Some readers may suffer from iatrogenic obesity. The word *iatrogenic* means that the condition is caused by medical treatment; in this case, by certain pharmaceutical agents. Of particular note to women is the well-known side effect of estrogen replacement therapy or birth control pills. A number of my counseling clients have experienced from fifteen to thirty pounds of immediate weight gain after going "on the pill." But estrogenic drugs are not the only drug-induced cause of weight gain, and while this topic is too large to be covered adequately in this context, here is a short list of prescription medications that are well known to cause weight challenges.

Prednisone

Acebutolol
(from fluid retention)

Astemizole

Atenolol
(from fluid retention)

Carbamazepine
(from fluid retention)

Chlorpromazine

Chlorpropamide

Clomipramine

Clonidine
(from fluid retention)

Dexamethasone

Diclofenac
(from fluid retention)

Diflunisal
(from fluid retention)

Diltiazem
(from fluid retention)

Doxepin

Enalapril
(from fluid retention)

Estrogens

Glipizide
(from fluid retention)

Ibuprofen
(from fluid retention)

Imipramine

Indomethacin
(from fluid retention)

Isradipine
(from fluid retention)

Ketoprofen
(from fluid retention)

Labetalol
(from fluid retention)

Lithium

Medroxyprogesterone

Methyldopa

Methylprednisolone

Minoxidil

Naproxen
(from fluid retention)

Nafarelin

Nortriptyline

Oral contraceptives

Perphenazine

Phenylbutazone

Piroxicam

Prochlorperazine

Tamoxifen

Thiothixene

Tolmetin
(from fluid retention)

Trifluoperazine

Verapamil
(from fluid retention)

This list is by no means exhaustive. If you are using a prescription medication and have experienced unexplained weight gain, ask your physician for recommendations. It is possible that she or he may be able to suggest an alternative medical treatment that will better accommodate your needs.

you may be genetically predisposed to weight gain

Do you have fat in your genes? Are your parents or grandparents heavy? When your family pulls together several generations of aunts, uncles, cousins, grandfolks, and miscellaneous other relatives for a family reunion, is the most striking cross-generational physical resemblance an expansive hip or waist girth? When you say you have a "large family," are you referring more to the physical size of the individual members than the extent of the family unit? Unfortunately, there is a genetic correlation between what Grandma weighed and what you weigh.

While it may be fashionable (and of questionable honesty) to lay the blame for all of life's ills at the feet of Mom and Dad, the genesis of excess fat goes beyond psychological fashion statements and is in a very real sense a genetic gift from your ancestors. Studies show that if your parents were heavy, you may very well be heavy, too.

An article appearing in the peer review journal *Metabolism* confirms the connection between genetics and weight problems. Predisposition to weight gain starts very early in life and is probably already entrenched from the moment of conception. A study done in 1976 on mice supports the notion that there is a metabolic difference between obese and lean mice, and while we certainly aren't mice, the metabolic similarities of mice and men can't be completely ignored.[2]

These mice were studied between the ages of seventeen days and eight weeks of age. By the age of four weeks, the obese mice already showed signs of altered weight, including elevated blood sugar and systemic insulin, obesity, reduced skeletal growth, and insulin resistance—differences that were unrelated to diet. All the mice in the study belonged to the same species of mice so their capacity to store fat, secrete insulin, and resist the effects of insulin were based on another genetic component. Fat was, literally, in their genes.[3]

Some of these issues of genetic tendency are too complicated to explore adequately in this context but there may be several faulty mechanisms at work here, including low thyroid function (a body-slowing trait that can be passed on generationally), inadequate levels or activity of brown adipose tissue, excessive production of insulin (or its counterpart, excessive sensitivity to carbohydrates), and others. We will deal with these issues in detail in later chapters.

When obese Zucker rats were studied to learn just why they were obese when their brothers, sisters, and cousins were thin, it was found that the tendency toward obesity was already evident within the first week of life. One article stated that "the main characteristics of the [obese Zucker rats] are hyperphagia [overeating], hyperinsulinemia [excessive levels of insulin in the blood stream], impaired thermogenic capacity [body temperatures were too low], high white adipose tissue lipoprotein lipase activity [increased tendency to store fat tissue], and a high rate of hepatic lipogenesis [liver producing too many fats]."[4]

Researchers forgave the little rats for overeating by saying,

> total additional energy consumed over the fifteen-week period cannot account for the greater body weight gain of the obese rats . . . the energy absorbed by the gainers was not significantly greater than that absorbed by the resisters or controls . . . that differences exist in the metabolic response to the purified moderately high fat diet . . . obesity prone individuals are more efficient than their leaner counterparts and thus utilize less energy per unit. . . .[5]

In other words, the obese rats gained weight not because they ate more but because their bodies were more efficient and required fewer calories to maintain core body activities than their lean counterparts. It had nothing to do with diet and everything to do with genetics.

Thankfully, we are not passive victims of our family tree. Although we may have to work a little harder than our lean human counterparts, we can unravel the genetic tangle by utilizing proper nutrition.

you may have been set up for obesity in childhood

Did yesterday's donut put the extra pound on your hips, or was it that donut you ate forty years ago? Or more accurately, was it those donuts and other sugary food artifacts you consumed throughout the first two decades of your development? How did eating habits in your formative years affect your tendency to gain weight now?

It is possible that poor dietary habits during those years when internal organs and body systems were being shaped have forever changed the way your body uses and stores energy. In other words, dietary indiscretions in childhood have damaged your homeostatic balance and possibly some key metabolic organs, and set you up for dietary challenge in adulthood.

Those of us who are now in our thirties, forties, and fifties grew up in the golden age of technology, especially food technology. No need to slave over a hot wood stove all day when you could pull dinner out of a box and set it steaming hot on the table within twenty minutes. Remember when TV dinners hit the market? How about instant mashed potatoes, Hamburger Helper,

SpaghettiOs, and Rice-A-Roni? If you were like me, lunch was Campbell's Chicken Noodle Soup, a glass of reconstituted powdered milk, and a peanut butter and jelly sandwich (Wonder Bread and Jiffy's, of course).

> *"I try not to eat things in public. I have to hide everything I do because I feel someone is going to think something."*
> **ALICE C.**

Sugar consumption increased exponentially in the fifties. You weren't eating breakfast if you weren't reading the back of a cereal box. The Pepsi generation came of age long before Madison Avenue called it that, with the per-person consumption of soft drinks increasing from over ten gallons in 1950 and over sixteen gallons in 1960, to nearly forty-seven gallons per year in 1993.[6]

During this period of increasing consumption of highly processed, highly sugared, highly artificial foods was a declining value in "natural foods." For example, my own dietary history is grim but typical for my generation. I grew up on a tiny farm in a remote part of the country. My mother raised virtually all our vegetables on her plot of garden. She purchased crates of fresh fruits and canned hundreds of jars of jams, jellies, fruits, and vegetables, which we enjoyed each winter and spring. Mom liked to bake bread. Since homemade bread was cheaper than commercially produced bread, she purchased white flour in hundred-pound cloth bags and kneaded and baked several loaves each week, which we ate dripping with homemade butter and jam.

Sounds idyllic doesn't it? But a closer look at that diet may explain the health challenges I now experience in my late forties. The homemade jams and jellies contained more sugar than berries and were cooked until every vitamin or mineral molecule had evaporated into the hot kitchen air. Mom's hobby of canning fruits and vegetables for the county fair was profitable. Every year she scored blue ribbons for her efforts. The prizes? Several hundred pounds of sugar and cases of Karo syrup. Our family of seven polished off every speck of sugar and every drop of Karo syrup before the next autumn fair rolled around. And that didn't count the sugared cereals, the carbonated drinks, the candy bars.

The result? A permanently disabled or exhausted pancreas, the very critical organ that regulates blood sugar by regulating the flow of insulin and glucagon and the secretion of digestive enzymes. This important system that pulls excess sugars out of the bloodstream simply wears out from overuse.

Mom isn't the only guilty party here. I have to take my share of the blame. After all, I *liked* the sugar and junk food! I ate it very willingly. And after I left home and started making my own dietary choices, I *chose* junk food. I ate out of cans, boxes, and packages. I patronized every fast-food establishment in a ten-mile radius and selected the worst that the good restaurants had to offer. Only when my health started failing in my twenties did I finally look at my diet.

No, actually, it was my brother who piqued my curiosity. One hot summer afternoon, I made a pitcher of iced tea and laced it with several scoops of sugar. My brother watched me stir in the sugar and quietly said, "Don't you know that sugar is a poison?" This simple question initiated my quest for better health through improved nutrition.

Some twenty years later, my health is better than it ever has been, but I still bear the scars of thirty years of abuse. And I probably always will. I am convinced that excessive sugar and rancid fat consumption during formative years taxes the ability of the pancreas to regulate blood sugars normally and sets us up for insulin resistance and carbohydrate sensitivity later in life. Both these conditions are directly linked to increased tendency toward weight challenges.

Our rat friends from the research labs have provided us with valuable information about the effect of childhood eating patterns on adult health problems. One group of rats was fed the ideal diet, according to most American children. During the first few weeks of life, they were fed a high-sugar diet, both by slurping it out of their feed bowl and having it injected into their veins. For a period of time, the high-sugar food didn't have an impact on serum insulin levels, but after eight weeks of the steady onslaught of sugar, the rats' defense mechanisms began to wear out and insulin poured into their blood in a desperate attempt to keep blood sugar under control. (More on why this is important in chapter 6.) The authors concluded "that long-term consumption of a diet in which available carbohydrate is rapidly absorbed causes insulin resistance in rats. The more rapidly that glucose is absorbed from the diet, the faster the insulin resistance develops."[7]

Keep in mind that insulin resistance developed primarily as a result of the fast absorption of the simple sugars. Complex carbohydrates found in fresh fruits and vegetables don't have the same quick, deleterious effect on insulin levels.

Another group of rats, however, were fed a diet that may more closely imitate that of our kids—high-sugar *and* high-fat foods. The deadly combination of the sugar and fat was devastating to their homeostatic mechanisms, both in raising insulin levels and

> *"My own diet is basically the
> starvation diet. I lost about
> thirty pounds, then said, 'To
> heck with this.' Starvation
> gets old real fast."*
> **FRANK**

reducing the ability of the body to transport the sugars through the bloodstream and deposit and use it appropriately.[8]

Unwittingly, our mothers may have made another "fatal" mistake in our infancy when they, under pressure from the doctor or the culture of the fifties, substituted breast milk with cow milk–based formulas. It is now well known that the consumption of cow's milk and other dairy products during the first year of life predisposes a child toward adult onset insulin-dependent diabetes by destroying beta cells in the pancreas, one of the major causes of obesity.[9]

Soy-based formulas may not be any better. Of course, our mothers were not aware of the health consequences of this "minor" food change. They just thought bottle-feeding would free up some of their time, and baby seemed to thrive. It was a matter of convenience. But baby's body knew and reacted against it with permanent damage to the pancreas, and increased the potential for dairy-related allergies as well.

Putting the risk of diabetes aside, there is some indication that consuming cow's milk during *any season* of life by numerous strains of rats "significantly increases carcass lipid content (the amount of fat on the body)." A synopsis of one study reads that "the obesity produced by the CM (condensed milk) diet in six strains was not due to hyperphagia (overeating). . . . Only one of the six . . . of the strains that increased adiposity on the CM diet consumed more energy (calories) than controls during the seven weeks of the experiment."[10]

Whether or not this study has a correlation to human beings is unclear. The study was done with high-fat condensed milk, which most of us do not drink. But those of us who were given sweetened condensed milk formulas in the first year of life may have been set up for weight challenges that will haunt us for many decades of life.

I got stuck with this challenge. Within three days of my birth, my mother became ill and was readmitted to the hospital with a life-threatening kidney infection. Instead of taking me to the hospital with her and allowing me to nurse even during her illness, my mother handed me over to my grandmother, who dutifully mixed condensed milk diluted with corn syrup, a few drops of liquid iron, and diluted it with water and fed me the formula out of the bottle. She was happy to do it, I'm sure. But that artificial formula wasn't good for my little body. My younger brothers were fed this same formula, which was popular during at least one generation of young children. What damage that formula has inflicted on a whole generation of children who now struggle with pancreas-related disorders such as diabetes, weight challenges, and allergies!

During the first two years of our lives, most of us ate far *more* than our share of processed sugars and fats and far *less* than our share of essential nutrients. Most of us poured cow's milk on our numerous bowls of sugary cereal and washed down Oreos or home-baked peanut butter cookies with a glass or two of the white stuff when we came home from school. These common childhood indulgences may have set us up for insulin resistance that renders our bodies incapable of either utilizing insulin properly or even balancing insulin secretion against glucagon secretion. Diets that are high in processed sugars have been clearly shown to produce insulin resistance. Cow's milk and harmful fats have shown the same result. When we adhere to this type of diet during the formative years of life, when our organs and tissues are developing, what happens to our ability to balance blood sugars later in life? Research literature is virtually silent on the subject.

My personal belief is that for many of us, blood sugar homeostatic mechanisms have been permanently, irreparably harmed because of childhood dietary indiscretions. If we are going to get both our blood sugar levels and our weight under control, we'll have to double up on our efforts to balance our diets appropriately, to choose a diet that balances proteins, carbohydrates, and fats in such a way that the excess secretion of insulin is not stimulated and that glucagon secretion and activation are encouraged. For many of us who really messed up our bodies during childhood, this is going to take enormous effort.

It isn't that we *can't* be thin now that the health and vitality of our pancreas and other organs are diminished. We've been handed a bigger challenge, and we just have to work harder at it.

how to overcome your unique challenges

The issues we've discussed in this chapter have far-reaching implications, not only in the difficult concepts behind them but more importantly in how we are actually going to resolve the issues in our own lives. And because I am both a nutritionist and a woman who has much of the same dietary history as the rest of the United States (with all the accompanying problems!), I know just how difficult it can be to make significant changes to eating habits that have developed over decades.

Spend a little time with each of the concepts to make sure you understand the issues involved, and then spend a little time planning how to ingrain new habits into your daily routine. Here is a step-by-step list of just how you can start incorporating these ideas into your lifestyle.

Clean out your refrigerator and cabinets by removing all nonfoods. If the waste worries you, consider how wasteful it's going to be if you eat all that junk! Remember, nonfoods are foodlike products that were synthesized in some chemist's lab! Here's a list of what to purge from your kitchen:

Carbonated beverages	Packaged cereals
Simulated fruit beverages	Processed sugars
Packaged foods (with the possible exception of a few canned specialty items)	All other convenience foods (Ouch! That one hurt, didn't it.)
Chips (potato and corn)	

The only exceptions I make to this rule are a tiny amount of specialty pasta products (rice noodles, corn spaghetti) for an infrequent treat; certain high-quality bean or vegetable soups (for a quick emergency meal); and a few condiments like catsup, mustard, and soy sauce.

I allow my kids who are not struggling with weight issues an occasional bowl of cereal, but the family rule is that it contain no wheat or corn and less than 4 grams of sugar per serving. That may seem generous until you discover how few cereals fulfill those requirements. (I personally eat cereal only once every two or three months and find I don't miss it.)

While these changes may seem drastic, if you are struggling with weight issues or other health challenges that are seemingly unresolvable, you will notice an almost immediate benefit from taking these few steps. If you feel you just can't do it all at once, resolve to make one change per week and be faithful with each one until the new eating habits are in place. Most people find that once they adapt to a healthier lifestyle, they really don't want to regress!

So what *are* you going to eat now that you've cleaned out the pantry? Stock your refrigerator with fresh vegetables and moderate amounts of fruits. Snack foods may include celery stuffed with almond butter or toasted pumpkin or sunflower seeds. We'll cover more of what you *can* eat in a later chapter. Just be patient!

Eliminate all potential allergens from your diet. Here's another ouch! To refresh your memory, remember that the foods you eat most frequently or the foods to which you are addicted are the foods that are the likeliest to produce an allergic response, including weight gain. The most common allergens in the American diet are corn, dairy products, wheat and other grains, peanuts, chocolate, citrus, eggs, and to a lesser degree, soy. If you have already cleaned out your pantry, chances are good that you've eliminated many of these foods already, but take another look.

Any food can create an allergy problem. You may not be able to tell without the aid of a test which foods are problematic for you. I highly recommend that you ask your doctor for an allergy test that tests for IgG immune response.

You will need to eliminate these foods *totally* from your diet for at least six weeks before noticing any benefit. If you are only slightly allergic, you may be able to tolerate these foods occasionally and in small amounts, but I encourage you to keep your diet as clean of allergy-producing foods as possible.

Resolve your constipation and increase the health of your colon and intestinal tract by drinking eight to ten glasses of water per day and including lots of fiber-rich foods in your diet. You require from thirty to thirty-five grams of fiber per day; the average American eats less than ten grams per day. I suggest that you use a sugar-free fiber supplement to guarantee your intake of fiber. Check with your local health food store for a brand and type of fiber supplement that will accommodate your needs. Some fiber supplements are powdered; you will need to stir them rapidly into a large glass of water and drink immediately. Other supplements are in capsule or tablet form. Choose the one that works best for you, and be sure to drink lots of water.

One more suggestion regarding fiber supplements: If your body is unaccustomed to eating lots of fiber, start slowly. Gradually increase the amount of beans and vegetables each day. If you are using a fiber supplement, start with a lower dose and increase incrementally until you are at a dosage that is comfortable for you. To ignore this rule may invite intestinal discomfort at the very least and intestinal blockage at the very worst!

If you have increased the water and fiber to optimum levels and you are still not enjoying frequent, regular bowel movements, ask your local health food store for their recommendation on an herbal laxative. Avoid products that contain senna, and choose only moderate amounts of cascara sagrada. Senna can be habit-forming, can cause lifelong dependence, and can induce uncomfortable cramping as well. Cascara sagrada can also become habit-forming if used too frequently or in doses that are too high.

Some excellent suggestions for herbal laxatives include the Health Haus Kleen Tea, Nature's Way Naturalax Extra Strength #3, American Health Tam, Nutrition Now Fiberdophilus, Planetary Formulas Triphala, and Nature's Herbs LB. For an excellent combination of fiber and herbal laxative, Nature's Secret is a good choice (one of my favorites). For availability of any of these products, call one of the numbers in Appendix C or visit your local health food store or GNC.

Strengthen your pancreas and other digestive organs by using herbs and nutrients that nourish these organs. A number of traditional herbal/nutrient blends are marketed just for this purpose. Many of the herbs that stimulate digestion (like dandelion root, gentian, and ginger) are called "bitters."

Other digestive aids include the use of enzymes. Some excellent formulas include Enzymatic Therapy MegaZyme, PREVAIL Digestive Formula, Enzymatic Therapy ProGestAid, Eclectic Institute Neutralizing Cordial, Swedish Bitters, or the stimulating herbs dandelion and ginger.

Check with your local health food store or call one of the numbers in Appendix C for information on how to obtain these products.

are your hormones sending the right messages?

We've seen how important it is to deal with lifestyle issues that influence weight management, but we're going to have to dig deeper if we want to solve the problem of stubborn obesity for many men and women. We're going to have to gain insight into the role of the endocrine system and its hormones if we're going to bring our bodies back into homeostasis, back into weight balance.

Key regulatory organs of the endocrine system may be sabotaging your efforts to lose weight, no matter how carefully you balance your diet. If your body—through the endocrine sys-

Most aspects of body function are regulated and controlled by the organs of the endocrine system, which include the brain (particularly the hypothalamus), the pituitary gland, the thyroid gland, the parathyroid glands, the parafollicular cells, the adrenal glands, the pancreas, the gonads, the pineal gland, and the thymus. The gastrointestinal tract and the kidneys also have some endocrine functions.

The endocrine system maintains homeostasis, helping the body adapt to changes in both the external and internal environment. The endocrine glands do this via secretions of chemicals or hormones, which are released into the bloodstream and sent to various receptor sites throughout the body to affect the desired changes.[11]

tem—is sending the right messages, it will be a lot easier to get your diet under control.

Let's look at the endocrine messengers (or hormones) one by one to see how they affect weight management; then we'll see how to bring these hormones back into balance.

The Little
Giant
That Fell
Asleep

4

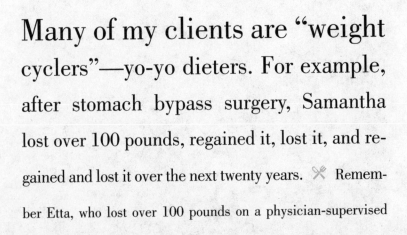

Many of my clients are "weight cyclers"—yo-yo dieters. For example, after stomach bypass surgery, Samantha lost over 100 pounds, regained it, lost it, and regained and lost it over the next twenty years. Remember Etta, who lost over 100 pounds on a physician-supervised liquid fast? She didn't eat a bite of real food for over a year. The moment real food reached her lips, it found its way back onto her hips. She regained all the weight she had lost, plus a little extra for good measure.

When I started helping Samantha and Etta with their eating plans, I said to myself, "They're going to drop the weight, and I'm going to be a hero! They'll love me for this . . ." And just as I hoped, the weight started to come off. The first week Samantha lost a few pounds, and so did Etta.

Over the next several weeks, both women continued to lose weight, slowly but surely. We laughed together with delight when they complained about their shoes flopping because their feet were shrinking. How fun it was!

And then, how abruptly it ended.

When Samantha and Etta had dropped thirty pounds, all weight loss stopped as if they had hit a brick wall. Samantha's uncontrollable cravings for chocolate returned with a vengeance, so I manipulated her diet a little more. I added some protein; I took away some calories. I added some carbohydrates; I dropped some carbohydrates. I did allergy testing and removed all offending foods from her diet (which included nearly everything she was eating). I increased both women's exercise programs. I told them to forget about the scales and try to relax. In short, I used every known theory to jar their bodies back into the weight-loss mode. Nothing worked. In fact, on less than 1,000 calories per day, Samantha gained back fifteen pounds. We all got a little desperate.

As I talked with other clinicians, I found out that Samantha's and Etta's experiences were not uncommon. For the truly obese, those over 120 percent of ideal weight, thirty pounds seems to be the "magic" number. They drop thirty pounds, and the body reacts by shutting down its ability to lose weight. Frustration and anger set in.

hypothyroidism, the underlying issue

If you're a carpenter, everything looks like it needs a nail. When you're a nutritionist, it seems as though every problem can be solved by tossing a salad at it. But those of us in the nutrition business have to realize that sometimes the problem may not be diet related. Other issues may be involved in weight control. And this is where most diet programs fall apart. They don't take into account the incredible complexity of the body. As I've already pointed out, unless the body's internal regulatory mechanisms are working correctly, all the diet modifications in the world won't work. You have to fix the underlying problem. In fact, the diet itself may create the problem.

Diets that are too low in fat; too high in highly processed fats; too high in refined carbohydrates; too low in complex carbohydrates; too low in protein; deficient in iodine, magnesium, zinc, chromium, or vanadium; too low in water; too high in thyroid-suppressing foods like cabbage or kale (an unlikely situation!); or too high in plant estrogens like soy protein powders all help to suppress the metabolic rate and make the body run slower, that is, more efficiently, on fewer calories. If this is your situation, you may lose a few pounds at the beginning, but suddenly all weight loss comes to a grinding halt. Why? Because you've begun to pull down the energy-producing giant of your body's own metabolism—the thyroid gland.

Tell your friends you're overweight because of "glandular problems" and you'll hear them chuckle behind your back: "She just needs to push herself away from the table." Now, even health professionals are beginning to see that a dysfunctional thyroid is indeed an issue with great numbers of Americans. Weight gain is only one side effect of *hypothyroidism*, the word we use to describe low thyroid activity.

> *"I gave my clothes to my dad*
> *and laughed. I can cheat*
> *once in a while and not feel*
> *guilty. I'll never gain the*
> *weight back again because*
> *I'm in control."*
> **JOHN**

The tiny thyroid gland has an enormous impact on the rest of the body. It is truly a giant in terms of influence; the cascade of biochemical events that creates this influence is both complex and fascinating. It doesn't actually start with the thyroid, however. The thyroid is Upper Management in terms of body organization. The thyroid is the Vice President of Operations, controlling the rest of the body upon orders from the top—the pituitary gland—which takes its orders from the hypothalamus, an even tinier organ nestled deep inside the brain at Corporate Headquarters.

The cascade of hormonal events starts with the hypothalamus, an endocrine organ located in the bottom portion of the brain, and leads to the stimulation of thyroid hormones in peripheral cells throughout the body. When blood thyroid hormone levels drop, the hypothalamus secretes TRH (thyrotropin releasing hormone), which signals the pituitary gland to secrete TSH (thyroid stimulating hormone). TSH enters the bloodstream, travels to the thyroid gland, and stimulates it to produce thyroxine (T4), a biologically inactive thyroid hormone which is then converted by an enzyme 5'-deiodinase into the biologically active thyroid hormone T3 (liothyronine). Partial T3 conversion takes place inside the thyroid gland, but primarily it takes place within cells throughout the body.

As T3 circulates through the bloodstream, it attaches to and enters cells via receptor sites on the cell membrane. Once inside, T3 increases each cell's metabolic rate, including body temperature, and arouses the cells to high anabolic (building) activity, stimulating the production of over 300,000 different protein bodies, such as hormones, enzymes, neurotransmitters, and muscle tissue. T3 also increases the utilization of oxygen and the excretion of carbon dioxide, a process that favors high metabolic activity. The active thyroid hormone is critical to an efficient, high-energy body.

In short, thyroid hormones control metabolism—the total of all processes involved in keeping the body alive and energized. It includes both anabolic (building) and catabolic (breakdown) processes.[1] Both anabolic and catabolic functions are critically and equally important, and both require energy. The amount of energy available to do these tasks is governed by the thyroid gland, or more accurately, by the hormones produced by the thyroid gland and received into the cell.

Each tier in the three-step process involved in thyroid function needs to be operative if the thyroid hormone is to effectively govern the body's metabolism—the initial production of T4, the conversion of T4 to T3, and the uptake of T3 through the cell wall. Any of these steps can malfunction for reasons including calorie restricted diets, systemic illness, certain medications, or selenium deficiency, which results in lowered metabolic rate and hypothyroidism, or other nutrient deficiences.[2]

HOW BODY TEMPERATURE AFFECTS THYROID FUNCTION

Clinical hypothyroidism is called myxedema. Symptoms of myxedema include a slowed heart rate; low body temperature;

sensitivity to cold; hypersensitivity to narcotics, barbiturates, and anesthetics; dry hair and skin; muscular weakness; depression; and not surprisingly, the tendency to gain weight.

If an individual recognizes himself in this clinical picture and asks his physician for a diagnosis, the physician will order a blood test that measures serum levels of T4 and T3 in the blood. This is where some of the confusion begins with the diagnosis of hypothyroidism. Serum T3 levels may not be a good way to test thyroid hormone levels.[3] Many doctors are beginning to believe that blood tests may have little to do with the efficiency with which T4 is converted to the active thyroid hormone T3, or with T3's uptake through the cell membrane and into the cell itself. Whereas relatively few people may be officially diagnosed with myxedema or hypothyroidism based on blood work or clinical observation, some clinicians have cited figures for subclinical hypothyroidism (not detected by the usual clinical tests) that range from 10 percent to 40 percent of the American population. Low thyroid function may not be readily apparent in these individuals through blood tests, but they may be experiencing the frustrating constellation of symptoms that portray a slightly dysfunctional thyroid gland.[4]

It simply may not be adequate to test thyroid function through a blood test if the activity of the hormone takes place within the cell instead of the blood. We may need to look at symptoms that include, in addition to those listed above, low blood sugar; weakness; dry, coarse skin; lethargy; slow speech; and swelling of face and eyelids. But the most telling symptom of low thyroid may be body temperature.

According to Dr. Broda Barnes, a medical doctor who devoted years of his life to the study of the thyroid gland, the most reliable indicator of thyroid function is the basal temperature test. He believes hypothyroidism is a major health concern in this country and that many disease conditions, including the tendency to retain excess weight, can be directly laid at the feet of this one fairly simple health challenge.

how to take your basal temperature

Shake down a basal mercury thermometer and leave it on your nightstand when you go to bed. For three consecutive mornings, before you get out of bed, place the thermometer in the base of your armpit and hold your arm close to your body. Keep the thermometer there for ten minutes. Write down your temperature each morning. (Women, ovulation can affect basal temperature, so the best time to do this test is on the second, third, and fourth day of your menstrual cycle. If you are no longer ovulating, you can do the test at any time. If you have a low-grade fever or are suffering from a cold or any other illness that could temporarily elevate your temperature, postpone testing until you are well.)

Normal underarm temperatures upon awakening range from 97.7 to 98.2 degrees. If the temperature is in the 97.2 to 97.7 degree range, the thyroid function may or may not be low. Check with your physician. Below 97.2 degrees, you will almost always experience additional symptoms and will need to be monitored and treated by your physician.[5]

One of the most fascinating books I have read on the subject of thyroid insufficiency was written by E. Denis Wilson, a medical doctor who coined a new phrase for subclinical hypothyroidism. He calls it "Wilson's Syndrome" (not to be confused with Wilson's Disease, which is a disease of copper metabolism). A syndrome is a cluster of symptoms that occur together and may be related to some type of biological dysfunction, in this case, thyroid enzyme dysfunction.

Dr. Wilson, author of *Wilson's Syndrome: The Miracle of Feeling Well*, considers the use of the early-morning temperature inadequate because the body's temperature naturally drops in the night to its lowest levels and may not rise to "normal" levels until three hours after awakening. He counsels patients to take their oral temperature three hours after waking and every three hours throughout the day. Oral *daytime* temperatures that average much below 98.6 degrees are problematic for the body, because low internal temperatures slow down the activity of the thousands of enzymes that are critically important for every chemical reaction that occurs in the body. It's easy to understand, given this model, the endless varieties of ways that hypothyroidism could have a negative impact on the body.

Dr. Wilson's list of symptoms of lowered thyroid *hormone* activity is so extensive that it ostensibly could include just about everyone. Where Dr. Wilson differs from many other practitioners is that weight management isn't high on his list. But the cluster of symptoms connected with Wilson's Syndrome may sound familiar to many people struggling with unresolved weight issues.

Fatigue	Decreased memory or concentration
Headaches, including migraines	Insomnia and narcolepsy
Premenstrual syndrome (PMS)	Anxiety and panic attacks
Irritability	Heat and/or cold intolerance
Dry hair or hair loss	Depression

Fluid retention

Inappropriate weight gain

Constipation and irritable
bowel syndrome

Dry skin

Allergies

Asthma

Itchiness

Hives

Unhealthy nails

Acid indigestion

Decreased motivation
and ambition

Decreased sex drive

Anhedonia
(decreased ability to enjoy life)

Irregular period
and menstrual cramps

Infertility

Decreased self-esteem

Decreased wound healing

Increased skin infections

Acne

Hemorrhoids

Hypoglycemia

Low blood pressure

Food cravings

Increased postprandial
response (fatigue or sleepiness
following a large meal)

Elevated cholesterol levels

Recurrent infections

Carpal tunnel syndrome

Lightheadedness

Dry eyes/blurred vision

Psoriasis

Changes in skin
and hair pigmentation

Flushing

Arthritis and muscular joint
aches, including fibromyalgia

Increased bruising

Musculoskeletal strains

Ringing in the ears

Abnormal throat and
swallowing sensations

Canker sores

Bad breath

Inhibited sexual development

Cold hands and feet, including
Raynaud's Phenomenon

Lack of coordination

Food intolerances

Abnormal sweating
(either decreased or increased
sweating)

Increased susceptibility
to substance abuse

This list includes so many body parts and functions that it seems unlikely so many disparate conditions could be attributed to one problem—low thyroid function. But the issue with the thyroid can be explained by that one phrase, "low body temperature" (resulting from low thyroid function).

THE ROLE OF ENZYMES IN THYROID FUNCTION

Let's jump for a moment to the subject of enzymes, the "workers" or catalysts of the body. Without enzymes, life ceases.

House construction provides a good analogy of the importance of enzymes. After an architect draws up house plans that detail every element of the dwelling, the building materials are purchased, including lumber, Sheetrock, plaster, plumbing fixtures, electrical wiring, paint, nails, screws, and hundreds of other items. All these raw materials just sit in a pile on the ground until the workers start putting the materials together according to the blueprint drawn by the architect.

Construction workers use the building materials to erect the house, but they are not altered by their work. After they have finished the house, they go to work on their next job, and so on.

In the body, the architect is the DNA/RNA code, and the construction workers are the enzymes. The materials they use include amino acids, vitamins, minerals, and other auxiliary substances. But the enzymes themselves remain unchanged by either the materials or the process. Without them, the body is inert, unable to complete any chemical process. As the enzymes energize these chemical reactions, they are reused by the body over and over again.

> *"After going through so many weight-loss programs and not being able to lose weight, I felt that I didn't even want to live. I was so depressed. Thank you, Carol! I've lost over thirty-five pounds and feel wonderful!"*
> JANE

Just as construction workers may enjoy certain working conditions, such as sunshine, regular meals, and a steady paycheck, your enzymes prefer certain conditions. High on their list is a body temperature of 98.6 degrees. When body temperatures drop drastically due to exposure to severe weather conditions, or when they elevate because of fever, many of the enzyme systems cease functioning. If the condition persists, permanent damage follows.

What happens in the event of slightly diminished body temperature? For example, what happens to the person who consistently runs a "normal" body temperature of 97.5 or 96.8 degrees caused by inadequate stimulation of the thyroid hormone on the cell? This condition isn't likely to destroy enzyme activity altogether. Dr. Wilson's position is that these subnormal temperatures simply slow down enzymatic reactions in the body, thus producing the wide-ranging symptoms listed above. He calls this Multiple Enzyme Dysfunction (MED), caused by inadequate conversion of T4 to T3 or insufficient uptake of T3 into cell structures. Without the stimulating effect of the thyroid hormone, body temperatures drop below the optimum 98.6 degrees.

One would think that if the thyroid malfunctioned at the same time that excess weight started piling on, weight-loss success would immediately follow resolution of the thyroid difficulty. However, this conclusion cannot be clinically predicted. In a telephone interview, Dr. Wilson related that weight issues may or may not be resolved simply by increasing body temperature or by increasing thyroid activity. The good news about resolving the thyroid issue is that your long list of thyroid symptoms, outside of the weight gain, can go away and you'll feel better! That's important, regardless of those few extra pounds of fat that may be more of a cosmetic issue than a health issue.[6]

If a sluggish thyroid truly is contributing to your weight gain, you will typically lose about fifteen to twenty pounds after correcting for thyroid deficiencies.

MINERAL DEPRIVATION

It has been estimated that up to 40 percent of our population suffers from subclinical hypothyroidism. If this is true, how did the thyroid get to be such a problem?

Possibly a number of factors in our culturally rich but nutritionally deprived culture slow down the organ that sits so high in the body's hierarchy of authority. Nutrient deficiencies in such important minerals as zinc and selenium are well known to produce low secretions of T3, the most biologically significant of the thyroid hormones. Selenium is a powerful antioxidant micromineral that is no longer found in the soil in many parts of the world, so food plants grown in the soil are deprived as well. As we eat less red meat, the richest source of zinc (other than oysters), we are becoming increasingly deficient in this powerful nutrient as well. Low zinc levels suppress thyroid function.[7]

High doses of ferrous sulfate (iron sulfate) significantly decrease thyroid hormone production so quickly that it becomes clinically detectable after just a few weeks.[8] If you need an iron supplement, you may prefer a less irritating form of supplementary iron, such as iron glycinate or an amino acid chelate taken simultaneously with vitamin C for maximum absorption. This source of iron should not suppress thyroid function. (Iron should be taken in small doses—up to 15 milligrams a day—and only after true iron-deficiency anemia has been diagnosed by the health care provider.)

IODINE GLUTTONY

Iodine is the most critical element in the thyroid hormone itself. The body contains about 25 milligrams of iodine, 20 percent of which is in the thyroid. According to Elson Haas, author of *Staying Healthy with Nutrition*, the concentration of iodine in the thyroid gland is more than one thousand times that found in the muscle. Approximately one-fourth of the body's supply of iodine is found in T4 and T3. Thyroxine (T4) is nearly two-thirds iodine. So we see the importance of this trace mineral in the production of these critical hormones.

The best source of organic iodine is the consumption of sea vegetables such as kelp. A diet rich in these foods could supply the body with sufficient quantities and the right type of iodine to supply the thyroid.[9]

However, in an attempt to go one up on nature and reduce the incidence of goiter (an enlargement of the thyroid gland caused by iodine deficiency, leading to hypothyroidism) in the central sections of the United States, *inorganic* iodine was added to table salt and by 1940 was in general use throughout the United States. While iodized salt may have solved some of the problems of iodine deficiency, such as goiter and cretinism that are epidemic in some parts of the world, it may have caused its own share of problems with the thyroid, including—you guessed it—hypothyroidism. In other words, both a deficiency and an excess of inorganic iodine causes thyroid deficiency!

Hand in hand with increased incidence of thyroid disease is an enormous increase in the consumption of iodine.[10] We only need about 100 micrograms per day of iodine, but Dr. Ross I. McDougall estimates that Americans consume from three to five times the amount required to sustain a healthy thyroid gland, well in excess of 500 micrograms of iodine per day.

> *"This was the easiest weight-loss program I've ever gone on. Even though I can't cook, I found I could follow these recipes. Even my friends can't believe I'm actually making gourmet diet food!"*
> **SANDRA**

With the extended and excessive consumption of salted foods, junk foods from fast-food chains, and salty snack foods, we are consuming enormous amounts of salt, most of which is laced with huge amounts of inorganic iodine, certainly enough to weaken the vitality of the thyroid. The iodized salt we're encouraged to purchase contains potassium iodide: inorganic iodine. One gram of salt contains about 76 micrograms of iodine, and the average person consumes at least three grams of salt per day, exceeding by over one-third the amount needed to produce thyroid hormone. If the iodine in the salt were organic, thyroid hormones would receive the iodine they need to synthesize the iodine within the hormone. But who knows the effect of these large quantities of inorganic iodine on our bodies? Could it be causing subclinical hypothyroidism?

Dr. Haas writes that "excessive quantities of iodized salt, taking too many kelp tablets, or overuse of potassium iodide expectorants such as SSKI can cause some problems, but regular elevated intake of iodine is needed to produce toxicity."[11]

Parenthetically, Dr. Haas notes that "goitrogens are substances that can induce goiter, primarily by interfering with the formation and function of thyroglobulin. Some natural goitrogens are soybeans, cabbage, cauliflower, and peanuts, especially when they come from iodine-deficient soils. Millet has recently been described as having goitrogenic tendencies."[12]

This isn't good news for diet-conscious vegetarians! More frightening, however, is the effect of both low-level radiation and high-level radiation on the thyroid gland.

RADIATION OVERLOAD

It took years for one of my colleagues who suffered from low energy, low body temperature, and other symptoms of hypothyroidism to discover that her thyroid gland was weakened. She recalled her teenage years when she received acne treatments. Every week her entire face, neck, chest, and back areas were bombarded with radiation. Of course, her thyroid gland was irradiated along with her face. Now she's dependent on supplemental thyroid hormone treatment to compensate for the damage done so many years ago in the course of "standard medical treatment."

How many full sets of dental X rays did we receive as children, with no protection offered to the thyroid area? In the fifties, the levels of radiation in dental X rays were many times higher than they are today. Combine frequent dental X rays with radiation released during testing in the forties and fifties from the nuclear industry, X rays from television sets that were much higher in radiation in that era, and the low-level radiation to which we are all exposed today, and it's easy to see that many of us are at high risk for thyroid dysfunction.

Current levels of radiation are increasing year after year, and we seem content to accept this environmental anomaly because we enjoy so many of the benefits that radioactive conveniences offer. After all, could we give up our cell phones, microwaves, and computers for the sake of health issues?

> *"If anybody tells you they can't succeed on this program, they haven't tried! Carol's program is so easy, it makes so much sense, and my body feels so good on it that there is no excuse for failure. I will never go back to my old way of eating."*
>
> **KAREN**

Several years ago documents released by the United States government showed that between 1944 and 1947, 400,000 curies of radioactive iodine were deliberately released into the atmosphere. (This is about 26,000 times more radiation than the radiation released in the Three Mile accident in 1979.) That particular government experiment will cost thousands of people their lives due to increased incidence of cancer, but the effect on the thyroid glands of possibly hundreds of thousands of people exposed during that time period may never be known.[13] We simply know that radiation exposure damages thyroid function, possibly beyond its ability to recover.

In his book *Solved: The Riddle of Illness,* Dr. Stephen Langer lists other possible causes of pandemic subclinical hypothyroidism, including the following:

Environmental pollutants in drinking water

Fluoride (particularly in low-iodine regions)

Certain prescription drugs (barbiturates, sulfa drugs, antidiabetic agents, synthetic estrogen, cough medicines, aspirin, and other salicylates)

Oil of wintergreen used in rubbing liniments

Cigarette smoke

Excessive intake of foods from the brassica family (cabbage, cauliflower, kale, turnips, mustard greens)

Excessive consumption of soy products, millet, and walnuts[14]

Regarding the impact low thyroid has on weight control, Dr. Langer further writes:

In order to be in good health and lose weight, you must have normal thyroid function—or appropriate supplementation—to realize full values from your food. Even if your diet contains all essential micronutrients (vitamins and minerals) in proper amounts, you may not be getting full nutritional benefit from it.

Food must be broken down and absorbed through the gastrointestinal mucosa. This process is often impaired in hypothyroidism. Next, food must be processed by pancreatic enzymes and converted by the liver in order to become biochemically active. Assimilation is often faulty in hypothyroid patients. Then the digested food must be transported by the circulatory system to the sites of use at the cellular level and successfully enter the cells to provide nutritional fuel. Lack of certain nutrients retards the process.

After all this, wastes have to be efficiently eliminated from cells and carried by the circulatory system for detoxification by the kidneys and liver and thrown off by the bowels, urinary system, skin, and lungs—all of which function below par in hypothyroid individuals.

In hypothyroidism, a decreased rate of oxygen use and a diminished rate of heat production translate into a decrease in metabolism and an inability to lose weight, no matter how hard we try. . . .[15]

Dr. Calvin Ezrin, author of *The Endocrine Control Diet*, states that low thyroid in itself does not necessarily cause obesity, a fact that is echoed by Dr. Langer. Langer reflected that about 40 percent of his hypothyroid patients are indeed underweight. But in the person already struggling with excessive weight, an underactive thyroid may make weight loss even more difficult to achieve, in much the way that your car just won't drive as fast if only one cylinder is firing.

Let's take a more in-depth look at the thyroid gland from the perspective of the yo-yo dieter.

linking yo-yo dieting and hypothyroidism

I took a trip to the university library and spent some time digging through medical periodicals on the subject of weight cycling, fully expecting to find reams of information on what happens to people who lose and regain weight over the course of a lifetime. The phenomenon is so common that I expected tons of research material, showing that the body actually begins to lose its ability to lose weight on any type of program because of reduced basal metabolic rate, which is governed by the thyroid gland. I already had a list of preconceived ideas about why this could happen:

1. The body's own homeostatic capabilities begin to break down from overuse.

2. Rebound dieters lose muscle tissue and gain fat during each cycle, depleting the amount of active tissue and making the body less metabolically active.

3. Inadequate protein intake or micronutrient deficiencies from inadequate consumption (the typical diet program) seriously erode the ability of the thyroid, pituitary, or other organs of the endocrine system to function normally.

4. The body's store of brown fat becomes incapable of burning calories efficiently, or the body loses its stores of brown fat because of frequent dieting.

5. The body refuses to lose weight after a period of deprivation. It instinctively knows that weight cycling is a risk factor for death and believes it is safer to be heavy than to continue cycling, so it just shuts down all weight-loss capabilities to save its life!

My list of theories was long—unlike the materials I found at the library. Even though a great deal of research has been done on obesity and many different weight issues, little has been done on the phenomenon of weight cycling. And what little research I did find was inconclusive and contradictory.

Let's look at some "cycling facts" from the perspective of the research community. An article in the *Journal of the American Medical Association (JAMA)* declares:

> There is no convincing evidence that weight cycling in humans has adverse effects on body composition, energy expenditure, risk factors for cardiovascular disease, or the effectiveness of future efforts at weight loss.
>
> The currently available evidence regarding increased morbidity and mortality with variation in body weight is not sufficiently compelling to override the potential benefits of moderate weight loss in significantly obese patients. Therefore, obese individuals should not allow concerns about hazards of weight cycling to deter them from efforts of controlling their body weight. . . .[16]

Other researchers agree that cycling does not have an impact on subsequent efforts to lose weight, citing possible compliance issues or metabolic changes. But when they addressed the issue of compliance, they wrote that "where compliance was consistent, weight loss was still significantly less on a second diet compared with the first." Some authors conceded that certain individuals may be susceptible or there may be "critical periods of vulnerability" where cycling does, in fact, shut down further weight loss.[17]

Conversely, an abstract from an article in *Archives of Internal Medicine* said:

> Repeated bouts of weight loss and regain, known as weight cycling or yo-yo dieting, are highly prevalent, occur in males and females, and are common in both overweight and

nonoverweight individuals. While there has been no consistent demonstration that, as was first thought, weight cycling makes subsequent weight loss more difficult or regain more rapid, it is possible that this does occur under some conditions or in particular individuals. There are stronger and more consistent links between body weight variability and negative health outcomes, particularly all-cause mortality and mortality from coronary heart disease. Weight cycling may also have negative psychological and behavioral consequences; studies have reported increased risk for psychopathology, life dissatisfaction, and binge eating. The bulk of epidemiologic research shows an association of weight variability with morbidity and mortality, although the mechanisms are not clear at present.[18]

We may not know exactly *why* weight cyclers suffer from health challenges, not the least of which is the inability to succeed on subsequent weight-loss programs, but studies clearly indicate that extremely low-calorie diets that are deficient in protein and carbohydrates slow down the metabolic rate by suppressing thyroid function, making it harder and harder to maintain normal weight, and harder and harder to maintain a healthy body overall.[19]

One author/clinician noted that if you're going to maintain your new weight level after following a restrictive diet, you must progressively keep dropping your calorie intake to accommodate your lowered metabolism (increased efficiency!) or you'll gain it all back. He also says that reduced weight comes along with side effects like hunger, cold intolerance, and just not feeling well. We've seen that these symptoms are typical of thyroid insufficiency.

Other medical journals say it "just ain't so!" They cite problems with the research.

Regardless of what the "experts" are saying, I still believe that when you significantly reduce the number of calories you eat on any type of a nutrient-restrictive diet, your basal metabolic rate drops and your body temperature decreases. I've seen it happen over and over again, as have other clinicians. You simply don't get as much heat production from burning those calories as

the thyroid and pregnancy

If you have given birth to at least one child, chances are good that your thyroid isn't working up to its potential. If you've given birth to several children, you can bet your bottom dollar that your body has slowed down! While part of your thyroid's laziness may be one of nature's secret birth control methods (hypothyroidism can cause reduced fertility), you may not necessarily appreciate nature's help. You may be able to control fertility without slowing down every other body function in the process and may not want the "help" of your thyroid.

Clinicians acknowledge that there is a spectrum of thyroid dysfunction in the postpartum period, but whether or not it is serious enough to qualify as clinical hypothyroidism (measurable by blood work) or is resolved over time is not certain.[21] Some authors have documented that symptoms of hypothyroidism can occur up to six months after the birth of the baby, but for some patients, it is never resolved. How many mothers are affected? Possibly up to thirty percent![22] For many of these women, the excess pounds accumulated during pregnancy will be nearly impossible to lose because of this reduced thyroid activity, regardless of diet or other lifestyle factors complicating an already complex gender-related weight issue.

you do on a higher-calorie diet. Your body becomes more efficient in converting that energy and storing it as cellular energy (fat tissue), and enzyme activity possibly diminishes. Both the thyroid and BAT are rendered helpless in the face of sluggish metabolism!

The good news is that a nutrient-dense, low-calorie diet may help prolong both your health and your life; in other words, you'll live slower but longer. The bad news is that if you ever start eating more calories, you body will label them "extra" and turn them into body fat, which is why the rebound effect in some people can be so powerful. You really do become an efficient fat-producing machine![20]

jump-starting the thyroid gland

Nutritionists have learned that regardless of what the research says, many people find it increasingly difficult to drop weight with each subsequent attempt. If you are going to lose weight (you will!) and keep it off (you can!), you're going to have to learn how to compensate for this new energy efficiency you've developed and trick your body into staying thin. For some people, that can be a real trick!

One study published in the *British Journal of Nutrition* had some good news, and we'll bring this information into our eating plan at the end of the book. Yes, reducing calorie intake may reduce the basal metabolic rate (BMR) of the body, but this isn't irreversible.[23] All you have to do to get your BMR back up again is to increase the number of calories you're eating. The trick is to do it without subsequent weight gain! We'll show you a way to increase your BMR and your calorie intake without regaining your weight. And you'll feel great doing it!

It may not be so important to know just *why* your thyroid

gland isn't functioning properly; that may be so much water under the bridge. It's more important to find out *if* your thyroid gland is functioning properly—if those all-important hormones are being actively used to their full potential. The easiest way to obtain this information is to do the basal temperature test described in this chapter. If your temperature is consistently more than two-tenths of a degree lower than 98.6 degrees, check with your physician for assistance in elevating your basal temperature. Treating thyroid insufficiency is not a do-it-yourself project.

I also recommend that you discontinue the use of commercially iodized salt (salt that contains potassium iodide). Use sea salt or kelp to season your food, and include generous amounts of seafood and sea vegetables in your diet. If possible, avoid the use of medications and the excessive consumption of foods that repress the natural vitality of the thyroid, such as Brussels sprouts, cabbage, and other brassicas, and soy foods.

The little giant that controls so much of our metabolism may not be to blame for *all* our weight troubles, but it may be part of the mystery that needs solving before we can lose the weight we need to lose.

Even if low thyroid function isn't causing your weight gain,

> *"After just six weeks on this program, my shoes are falling off my feet and I'm already out of my clothes. I just bought new sneakers and already they are too big for me. Help! I need new clothes!"*
> **PAT**

just getting your hormone levels up to where they should be will make you feel better. And who knows? If you're a little more active, maybe you'll end up doing a little more exercise!

Thyroid hormones aren't the only messengers that deliver faulty messages to the fat-regulating sensors of the body. If you're female, your chances of hormone-related weight challenges increase exponentially. And if that piece of news isn't enough to send you into a chocolate-eating binge, how about if you're forty or over and female?

Fat,
Frustrated,
Forty, and
Female

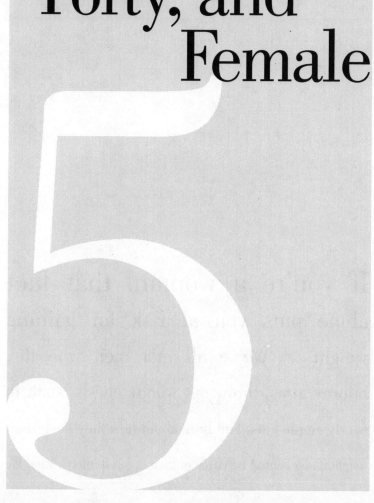

If you're a woman, that fact alone puts you at risk for gaining weight. ✂ We've all met men who flex brawny arms, throw out wimpy chests, suck in overly ample guts, and brag about how they keep their weight under control by virtue of their . . . well, their virtue. We see their wives or girlfriends smile politely and perhaps a little painfully. Most of those female counterparts who struggle to keep their weight under control would sell their souls to get a taste of that confident macho ego. They know how hard they fight the weight war—and they also know that, generally speaking, they watch what they eat infinitely more carefully than *he* ever did! It just doesn't seem fair. And it isn't.

While many men (the unenlightened ones) like to think their chubby wives just don't exhibit as much self-control as they do, the truth is, it's physically more difficult for women to lose weight. Female weight loss is simply not the same as male weight loss. While thyroid function plays a role (women experience hypothyroidism at a rate from five to ten times higher than men) the reason for this difficulty usually fits neatly into one word: hormones. Women have them; men don't—at least they don't have the hormones that affect keeping weight down. In fact, male hormones actually work *for* men while female hormones typically work *against* women. Men who enjoy high levels of testosterone (and what man doesn't?) also enjoy an increased metabolic rate and an increased tendency to build muscles, which, as we noted in chapter 4, helps keep the metabolic rate high.[1]

Men, if you are reading this book because you're the unfortunate half of the couple that struggles with weight, you'll love this book. Losing weight on a program of this type is much easier for you than it would be for the important woman in your life. You simply don't have as many issues to deal with. Women, keep reading. We'll resolve the issues for you as well.

According to studies dating back to 1976 and 1980, 25.7 percent of the population was overweight. More than nineteen million American women and fifteen million American men were affected. Over a ten-year period, the study showed that women gained more weight but men were at greater risk for *major* weight gain. The overall incidence of weight gain, however, was twice as great among females than males.

> *"Carol, thank you so much for writing this book. I've been using your program now for over a year and have lost over 100 pounds. My only question is, can you write some more recipes? This is the best food I've ever eaten."*
> —ANNE

Current data indicate that at any given time, one-third of American women and one-fourth of American men are trying to lose weight, and at least thirty-four million Americans are 20 percent or more overweight. This figure does not include many more millions of American women who struggle with that last fifteen to twenty pounds they can't seem to shake. There seems to be a complicated interconnection between hormones, mineral balances, and other factors that perplex an already complex issue for so many women. Getting those hormones to balance may be as difficult as balancing the national budget.

Pat's situation is typical of the struggles many women experience with weight. For the first twenty years or so, it wasn't difficult for her to keep her hourglass figure. But when the kids arrived and sent her hormones spiraling out of control, her concave figure turned convex. Suddenly "well rounded" didn't have anything to do with life interests.

While both of Pat's parents were heavy, and her father was an alcoholic, Pat was an athlete. She earned basketball scholarships and enjoyed power lifting. When she got married she weighed about 135 pounds. With the arrival of baby #1 came an additional sixty pounds that didn't disappear. She was at 220 pounds when she got pregnant the second time. From then on, the weight just piled on.

Pat's problem isn't that she eats differently than when she was an athlete or before the babies arrived. While her eating habits have never been terrific (she eats for comfort and to calm her nerves), her body doesn't deal with food as it did before. Her body has changed. Before she had children, her body burned the excess calories; now it stores them.

RIDING THE ESTROGEN/PROGESTERONE SEESAW

Whereas a man's body might be compared to an electric typewriter, a woman's body could be compared to an IBM PC. Women are complex creatures with parts and systems that don't always function well. Just experiencing monthly cycles with hormones that fluctuate on a regular basis is complicated enough. But when a woman becomes pregnant, hormones and nutrients set up an intricate game of seesaw that can continue for years after the pregnancy is over. With each subsequent pregnancy and birth, the game gets more and more convoluted until, after childbearing has ceased, the game doesn't end. The players don't seem to know when it's time to call it quits.

CONVERSATIONS BETWEEN THE THYROID AND THE OVARIES

The interconnection between these hormonal messengers is so complicated that we're tempted to throw up our hands and say, "I can't figure it out, so let's just get on with life." Let me try to simplify it for you.

First of all, thyroid hormones and female hormones "talk" to each other. David Watts, Ph.D., author of *Trace Elements and Other Essential Nutrients,* writes of the effect thyroid hormone has on estrogen production and, subsequently, on progesterone production, and vice versa. He says that estrogen dominance, either through oversecretion of the ovaries or through estrogen replacement therapy with synthetics, pulls down the function of the thyroid gland and the metabolic rate of the body, with symptoms ranging from weight gain, blood sugar disturbance, fatigue, and even depression.

> *"My friends keep saying, 'How did you lose all that weight?' But I promised not to share the recipes with anyone until the book came out. Please, Carol . . . I can't hold them off much longer! We need this book!"*
> **JUDY**

Progesterone, estrogen's complementary hormone, reverses this tendency, facilitating the functioning of the thyroid gland and possibly assisting in weight loss, reducing the tendency toward water retention, depression, low energy levels, and other symptoms.

We've seen the impact that pregnancy has on thyroid function. Up to 30 percent of women can experience either clinical or subclinical hypothyroidism after pregnancy, and the likelihood of developing low thyroid function increases with each subsequent birth. Sometimes these thyroid issues will resolve themselves. For large numbers of women, they will not be resolved without outside help.

During pregnancy, and in women using oral contraceptives, serum T3 levels decrease as thyroxine-binding globulin (TBG) increases, leaving less access of the activating thyroid hormone to the cells.[2] While balancing the thyroid is not necessarily the key to weight loss, especially weight loss greater than fifteen pounds, until both hormone and thyroid issues are looked at and addressed, losing weight on any type of program is difficult.

There are actually four players—two hormones and two minerals—sitting on this seesaw: estrogen and progesterone, copper and zinc. During pregnancy, blood estrogen levels soar, increasing many times higher than prepregnancy levels. Excess estrogen means excess water weight, because estrogen sequesters salt and salt sequesters water.

Estrogen may decrease bowel motility—it may cause constipation. Estrogen-induced constipation sets up a negative downward spiral. As estrogens are used, they are supposed to be excreted by the liver into the intestine for elimination from the body. If excess estrogens cause fecal material to sit in the colon for prolonged periods of time, these used estrogens are reabsorbed into circulation through the bloodstream and are reused, causing even higher levels of circulating estrogen.

There's even more bad news. Elevated estrogens cause fat to be deposited in the tissues. While a little roundness makes females look female, too much roundness makes them look fat![3] The fat men deposit around their waists and hips actually contains more of the enzymes involved in breaking down fat tissue for energy than are found in female fat tissue.

Estrogen wields a powerful influence on the type of fat deposited in a woman's body that promotes fat storage. As one au-

thor says, "The action of female hormone is directly in opposi-
tion to that of most thermogenic substances." In other words,
women have a more difficult time just burning stored calories in
the production of heat because of estrogen's influence.[4]

As if the subject of hormones weren't complicated enough,
hormones are strongly influenced by the balance of minerals in
the body. This is where the subject gets really technical. Americans are notoriously deficient in key minerals, which can create
hormonal havoc throughout the body. Mineral deficiencies can
also create food cravings and other symptoms to which women
are much more susceptible than men.

zinc deficiency and copper toxicity

Minerals and other micronutrients aren't often brought into a
discussion on weight loss, but they certainly should be. Nutritional balance between the micronutrients is the single most important factor in restoring and building health. Maintaining ideal
weight is just one aspect of being healthy, but deficiencies or tox-
icities in one or more nutrients will make it difficult to meet your
weight goals.

There are two minerals that both oppose and complement the
actions of each another. When they are unbalanced, as they often
are in women, the result can be impaired weight control. These
two minerals are copper and zinc.

We don't discuss copper very often, and yet copper toxicity,
particularly when accompanied by zinc deficiency, can significantly alter a woman's ability to maintain her weight. Nutritionists encounter many clients, particularly women and children,
with inadequate levels of zinc and excessive levels of copper.

Copper performs many important functions in the body, such
as taking part in certain immune functions and building strong

arteries. The problem is not copper itself; the problem is excess copper in relation to zinc. Food is perfectly balanced between these two minerals in about an 8:1 ratio. If diet were our only source of copper, the balance between these minerals would probably not be an issue.

Unfortunately, we're getting copper from other sources. Copper is added to animal feeds and sprayed on vegetables and grains to help prevent fungal and algae growth. Copper pipes are now used in most newer homes. Copper is used in many dental appliances, and sometimes in swimming pools to purify the water. Many women have been fitted with copper IUDs for birth control purposes. Commonly used prescription medications, like certain sedatives, tranquilizers, and psychotropics such as Thorazine, Librium, Tofranil, and Miltown, to name a few, can contribute to copper toxicity. Deficiencies in other important nutrients, such as the B complex and iron, also lead to elevated levels of copper.

Much of this excess copper would be excreted out of the body *if* the diet were adequate in zinc. Over the past several decades, dietary patterns and soil conditions have dropped zinc consumption down to less than half of what it should be. Many young women and children consume virtually no zinc at all in their diets, leaving them particularly vulnerable to copper toxicity.

Copper toxicity is known to suppress thyroid function in susceptible individuals through a number of mechanisms, but primarily by influencing two other critical hormones: insulin and estrogen.[5] We'll deal with insulin in chapter 6. Right now let's discuss estrogen.

THE DARK SIDE OF ESTROGEN

Monthly cycles, pregnancy, lactation, and menopause cause estrogen levels to swing upward, and copper increases along with the estrogen. Women who have used birth control pills for any length of time often experience elevated copper levels with typical symptoms of depression, frequent headaches, fatigue, constipation, emotional volatility, weight gain, and raging food cravings (particularly for sweets, breads, and pastas).[6]

In the last trimester of pregnancy, both copper and estrogen levels soar, but after the baby has been delivered, copper levels are supposed to level out to balance zinc to the natural 8:1 balance.

Estrogen's opposing hormone is progesterone, the hormone that helps sustain the pregnancy. Progesterone is an extremely beneficial hormone. Adequate levels of it increase body temperature, possibly increasing enzymatic activity. It increases thermogenesis, or the "wasting" of excess calories, helps calm the brain, and prepares the body for pregnancy.[7]

Upon withdrawal of progesterone (or upon an increase in estrogen), the mother goes into labor and delivers the child. If estrogen levels remain high because the woman's hormonal system has become unbalanced or because copper levels remain elevated, progesterone levels will remain low. Think of it as a double seesaw. When estrogen is high, progesterone is low; when copper is high, zinc is low.

> *"After I lose the weight, I want to be here for my children. I want to go hiking again, and do family things without feeling like I'm going to have a heart attack!"*
>
> **GRACE**

The opposite imbalance rarely occurs, since the American diet is deficient in zinc-rich foods—red meat, oysters, and other seafoods and greens. Because we don't eat many of these foods, the delicate balancing act never takes place. The game to see which can rise higher, estrogen or progesterone, copper or zinc, plays on and on. The result? Postpartum depression and all the symptoms mentioned above in regard to birth control pills, including increased weight.

Resolving the zinc and copper issue is not difficult. Simply increase the amount of zinc in the diet for a few months and the excess copper is typically chelated—washed out of the body. Zinc and copper levels then return to normal and relieve the symptoms caused by the imbalance. Resolving the estrogen/progesterone issue may not be so easy. Women need to work with a nutritionally aware physician for tips on balancing their female hormones through the use of herbs and natural hormones.

This is where real confusion and frustration sets in. Virtually every woman who opts for estrogen replacement therapy to balance these hormones experiences weight gain. No question about it. This gain can range anywhere from just a few excess pounds of water to over twenty pounds of excess water and fat. Natural hormone-balancing agents, such as herbs, do not have this weight-enhancing effect. While they may take a little longer to become therapeutic, they can work effectively in balancing the female system.

menopause and weight gain

Sally recalled exactly when she gained her most recent weight: "I gained after the hysterectomy and going on Premarin when I was forty-three years old. I ate just as carelessly prior to that but never carried extra weight. I was always thin."

According to *The Essential Guide to Prescription Drugs, 1992*, side effects of estrogenic drugs include fluid retention and weight gain, and they call these effects "natural, expected, and unavoidable."[8]

In her book *Super Nutrition for Menopause*, Ann Louise Gittleman writes:

> The preliminary results of a survey conducted by Judith Wurtman, Ph.D., Massachusetts Institute of Technology, seem to indicate that 65 to 75 percent of women involuntarily gain weight at menopause . . . and it appears that a slightly higher percentage of women on hormone therapy gained weight compared to those women who took no hormones. . . . Those extra pounds that show up at menopause may be due to a lack of progesterone and the consequent estrogen dominance. Estrogen that is not balanced by an adequate amount of progesterone causes weight gain. This is something farmers have known for years; that's why the synthetic estrogen hormone diethylstilbesterol (DES) is given to steers to fatten them up.
>
> Another reason for the weight gain is that during the first ten days to two weeks of our menstrual cycle, our bodies use up a substantial number of calories in the process of ovulation. So when we stop ovulating (enter menopause) we are left with extra calories, up to 300 daily in some cases, that are not begin [*sic*] burned. . . . Weight gain during and after menopause may also result from negative attitudes about aging and perceived loss of sexual attractiveness. Many of us choose to compensate for this perceived loss through food.[9]

Clinicians understand the connection between menopause and weight gain. Dan Mowrey, author of *Fat Management: The Thermogenic Factor* and the Director of Research for the American Phytotherapy Research Laboratory, stated in a telephone interview that of the hundreds of women they have counseled over the past five years, about 20 percent cannot drop the weight no matter what they do, and the vast majority of these women are using estrogen replacement therapy.

Imbalances in the female hormone system occur routinely around the time menopause starts, around the age of forty to forty-five. But there may be a number of reasons why menopause (whether natural menopause or forced menopause through hysterectomy) can put the pounds on. As we've already noted, excessive estrogen in relation to progesterone causes the body to sequester both water and fat. The other side of the coin is that excess body fat increases estrogen levels because fat produces small amounts of estrogen. Obesity, therefore, can aggravate hormone imbalances along with premenstrual and menopausal symptoms. Many women's estrogen levels soar upon the onset of the perimenopausal years.

Isn't that wonderful—even your body fat jumps into the fray! Let's take a look at the most abundant form of fat in the human body: triglycerides. Triglycerides are what we ignominiously call body fat or white adipose tissue (WAT).

ESTROGEN AND TRIGLYCERIDES

Estrogen excites the liver to produce more and more triglycerides (from dietary carbohydrates, by the way) like an efficient internal fat factory. According to Dr. Calvin Ezrin, M.D., author of *The Endocrine Control Diet,* estrogen increases the production of triglycerides at a rate that will not be reversed when estrogen therapy is withdrawn.[10]

But we also eat triglycerides. Triglycerides are dietary fat. Dietary triglycerides are transported through the blood via protein/fat complexes called chylomicrons and are removed from

are you an android or a gynoid?

Obese women produce excess estrogen, which has been shown to promote breast cancer. Obesity may be classified in the android form, which is weight gain in the upper body, abdomen, shoulders, and nape of the neck, and the gynoid form, which affects the lower body, or the thighs and buttocks. Android obesity is associated with more pronounced metabolic and hormonal abnormalities, longer menstrual cycles, and various diseases, such as diabetes. Women with android obesity have decreased levels of sex hormone–binding protein and increased levels of estrogen, which may increase their risk of breast cancer.

The influence of body fat distribution on breast cancer risk was assessed. Various body measurements, including height, weight, and thigh, abdomen, suprailiac (flank), waist, and hip circumferences, were made on 216 patients with breast cancer and 432 normal subjects. Patients with breast cancer had greater ratios of waist-to-hip circumference than normal subjects.

The risk of developing breast cancer increased with increasing ratios of waist-to-hip circumference and suprailiac-to-thigh skin fold. Patients with breast cancer also had greater upper body obesity, such as within the skin folds of the triceps and biceps. The results suggest that women with android obesity are at a high risk of developing breast cancer.

Studies indicate that fermented soy and soy products help reduce the risk of breast cancer. If you or a family member has a history of breast cancer or are at risk for developing breast cancer, speak with your health care professional about how to use soy to your advantage in your quest to avoid breast cancer yet not gain excess water weight while using it.[11]

the blood by an enzyme called lipoprotein lipase (LPL). LPL
pulls triglycerides into the adipose (fat) cell for storage. Guess
which powerful hormone stimulates the activity of LPL? That's
right. Estrogen stimulates the activity of LPL in certain regions
in the body, most notably the abdominal region.

Scientists have learned that LPL is increased during periods
of weight gain, in both obese and nonobese persons. However,
when a nonobese person loses excess weight, LPL returns to normal levels, shutting down the deposition of excess fat into adipose tissue. In the "reduced-obese" person, however, LPL does
not decrease and may actually increase, leading to *increased* and
easier weight gain. The difference, apparently, has nothing to do
with the diet of the obese or the nonobese individual. The difference is genetic. Genetically obese rats have characteristically
higher levels of LPL. (Incidentally, smoking stimulates LPL activity.)

High-fat diets (the greasy-hamburger-and-potato-chip variety) increase estrogen levels in the blood. Pesticides that contain
estrogenic chemicals disturb the delicate estrogen/progesterone
balance in both the female and male body, as can chemical
residues from plastic bottles that have leached into bottled water.

The overall message of estrogen as it relates to weight loss is
that if you are a woman in the age range between forty and sixty,
and are either in the middle of or have already passed through
menopause, you may gain an extra five to twenty-five pounds because of an estrogen/progesterone imbalance. As Dr. Ezrin
stated, these pounds are not necessarily *fat* but may be water due
to salt retention. The message is: Stop trying so hard to lose *fat*.
Instead, balance out estrogen levels by increasing the amount of
fiber in your diet (to about thirty-five grams per day), drink eight
to ten glasses of water per day, and avoid foods to which artificial
estrogens have been added (like nonorganic red meats and poultry). If your physician suggests it, use hormone-balancing herbs

or natural progesterone creams or natural hormone replacements that help to restore the female hormone balance to your body.

While all the information in this chapter may seem dauntingly difficult to assimilate and incorporate into your own health picture, just learning about how powerfully your hormones affect you is a big step toward getting your body weight back in control. You didn't get out of balance overnight, and you won't get back in balance overnight. But starting today, you're on your way to better health.

> *"You come to a moment in time where you realize that the decision to lose weight is there, and it is a mental decision. It is not 'Well, someday . . .' Today is the day I start! And that's it! You don't look back!"*
> **ESTHER**

There are two more sets of hormones that influence weight, probably in a more powerful way than either the thyroid hormones or the female hormones. While approximately 80 percent of overweight Americans suffer from an imbalance in these two hormones, the good news is that for the vast majority of people struggling with weight, these hormones are easily brought under control just by changing the composition of the diet. In other words, a properly balanced diet really can lead you in the direction of permanent weight maintenance. Let's take a look, now, at insulin and glucagon.

Squabbling
Sisters

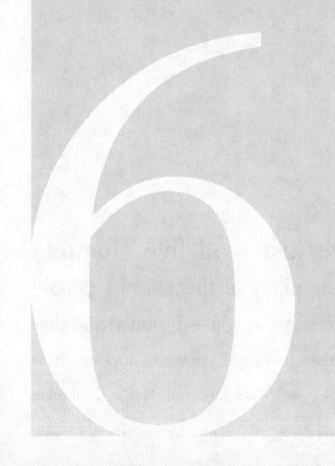

You've just read five chapters outlining many of the reasons people gain excessive weight—dysfunctional thyroid, female hormones, genetics, a dormant or lost BAT supply (brown fat). And there's no question that poor food choices, particularly our obsession with nonfoods, has driven our bodies over the brink of metabolic exhaustion. It's going to take more than wishful thinking or good intentions to get back on track with our health and our weight.

However, the most fundamental reason most of us wrestle with our weight is the imbalance of two critical hormones, *insulin* and *glucagon.* The pancreas secretes these hormones in response to the level of sugar in the blood. Insulin and glucagon regulate how much energy is used and burned and how much is stored as body fat. Like squabbling sisters, insulin or glucagon achieves ascendancy only at the expense of the other. When one is up, the other is down.

The principle here is simple: Excess carbohydrates stimulate the secretion of insulin, a fat-storing hormone. As insulin goes up, glucagon goes down and is not able to fulfill its role of pulling sugars and fats out of storage to spend them as energy in the brain and the rest of the body.

HOW WE ACCESS ENERGY

Even the thinnest of us have enormous stores of energy locked away in fat cells distributed throughout the body. It only remains to learn how this energy is accessed when the need arises. Let's look at the "Energy Accessibility Cycle" more closely.

After you eat a meal, the sugars in the meal are deposited in the bloodstream in the form of glucose. Glucose is the #1 source of energy to the brain; a constant supply is absolutely critical for brain function. When circulating levels of glucose get too high, insulin pulls the excess sugars out of the bloodstream and deposits them in the liver in the form of glycogen. When the liver reaches capacity, it turns the sugars into triglycerides and deposits them in fat tissue throughout the body.

When blood sugar levels get too low, glucagon reaches into the liver and pulls glycogen out of storage, converts it back into glucose, and allows it to circulate throughout the bloodstream. When glycogen runs low, triglycerides, or body fat, are converted back into glucose to bring circulating glucose levels back up to normal.

The secret to permanent weight loss is to encourage the body to keep sugar levels low, thereby suppressing the secretion of insulin and increasing the secretion of glucagon.

If you can appropriately balance insulin and glucagon every time you eat a meal, every time you put something in your mouth, you'll be able to control your weight almost without trying, for the rest of your life. Your hormones will work *for* you instead of *against* you! Most important, weight loss will be *fat* loss, not muscle or critical water supply. You won't feel hungry. You'll have lots of energy and you'll feel great.

Let's take a closer look at how insulin and glucagon wield such a powerful effect on the human body and its ability to stay thin.

blood sugar and the high carbohydrate diet

We must explore some fairly intricate hormonal issues if we want to understand the effects of a high-carbohydrate diet on insulin and glucagon ratios. While the body is blessed with an enormous capacity to maintain homeostasis in a very unbalanced world, its homeostatic mechanisms are not infinite. If we want to maintain homeostatic balance and thus keep our weight under control, we must learn how these unbalanced hormones cause weight gain and what we can do to stop their squabbling.

First of all, we need to understand how eating a diet high in carbohydrates affects blood sugar, because the secretion of insulin and glucagon is determined by the level of sugar in the blood.

Think about the source of carbohydrates. Foods like apples, carrots, pasta, cereals, potatoes, rice, baked beans, candy bars, potato chips, and soft drinks have at least one thing in common: They are sugars. Complex carbohydrates—raw fruits, grains, and vegetables—contain complex sugars called disaccharides or polysaccharides, two or more sugar molecules bound together by molecules of water.[1] Because these sugars are too large to be absorbed into the bloodstream and burned as energy, they must be digested into single molecules, or simple sugars, for conversion to blood sugar (glucose). The tough fibers encasing these molecules in complex carbohydrates are very beneficial to the body because they help sweep the intestinal tract clear of dietary debris, encourage the proliferation of friendly bacteria, lower blood fats, and eliminate used estrogens from the body.

On the other hand, simple carbohydrates like sucrose, honey, corn syrup, or white table sugar are tiny molecules that have been stripped of their natural fiber coating and can easily cross the intestinal barrier. They absorb quickly into the bloodstream. The sugars released from simple carbohydrates can be dumped into the body within seconds by absorption through the mucosal membrane of the mouth. (If you want to see how rapidly sugars can be absorbed, take a large sip of dinner wine and swish it around in your mouth. See how quickly you feel the effects of the alcohol, which is a sugar. You can feel it within seconds!)

Both simple and complex carbohydrates must be broken down into glucose to be used for the production of energy in the body. Let's follow these carbohydrates as they make their way through the intestinal tract to discover their final destination and what role they play in fat deposition.

The process of digestion begins in the mouth via amylase,

the carbohydrate-digesting enzyme secreted in saliva. The act of chewing exposes the food particles to the effects of the amylase, which starts to work immediately on the long-chain carbohydrates or sugars in the food. After you swallow food, it sits in the cardiac portion of the stomach for a few minutes, but that resting time is not wasted. While the food is heating up to 98.6 degrees (the temperature at which enzymes work most efficiently), the amylase continues to cleave the sugars into smaller and smaller units.

> *"Why did I eat it? Because it was in the kitchen! Why was it in the kitchen? Reality check!"*
> **CHRISTINE**

As the food passes through the small intestine, the final process of digestion takes place and the carbohydrates from your last meal are finally reduced to single molecules of glucose and received through the intestinal mucosa into your bloodstream.

Regardless of the original chemical composition and amount of fiber these sugars come wrapped in, a carbohydrate is still a sugar, and the digestive destination of either complex or simple carbohydrates is simple sugars, which are readily absorbed into the bloodstream. In a real sense, the body's response to simple sugars from cakes and candies is not very different from the complex sugars found in high-fiber vegetables and fruits because the result is the same—the production of glucose. Only the rate at which they are absorbed differs.

If we consider the diet plans of gurus like McDougall, Barnard, and the Diamonds, the enormous quantities of grains, vegetables, and fruits they recommend we consume are turned into large quantities of sugar that ultimately flood the intestine. This is where the critical hormones insulin and glucagon enter the picture. When sugar is absorbed into the bloodstream after a meal (particularly a meal high in carbohydrates) the pancreas squirts insulin into the bloodstream to compensate for the sudden onslaught of sugar, pulling the excess sugars into the liver and storing them as glycogen that can be released for energy later as the need arises. Glycogen is a ready source should you need quick energy.

When the liver's storage capacity is filled, the excess sugars are then deposited as fat tissue throughout the body. The body's ability to store excess carbohydrates as fats is virtually unlimited as new storage tanks—fat cells—can be built very quickly. Once built they remain forever, thus ensuring a ready site for fat deposition should the need arise at another time.

It's true that simple sugars absorb more quickly than complex sugars, creating a more volatile blood sugar/insulin reaction with more serious and long-term consequences to the body. But given the fact that all carbohydrates are digested down to simple sugars sooner or later, we have to understand that the ultimate fate of carbohydrates unopposed by the adequate consumption of proteins and fats is the release of insulin, the hormone that facilitates the storage of fat.

To make matters worse, every gram of glycogen stored in the liver is attached to three grams of water, making you pack on the water weight in addition to packing on the fat weight. That's probably why going on an insulin-reducing diet causes an immediate loss of about ten to fifteen pounds in the form of water.[2]

WHY GLUCAGON IS YOUR FRIEND

Glucagon, the more obscure of the hormonal sisters, is the dieter's friend. Glucagon is a protein molecule made up of a configuration of twenty-nine amino acids, including threonine, methionine, leucine, tryptophan, glycine, valine, tyrosine, and other essential and nonessential amino acids. (Vegetarian diets are low in some of these critical amino acids.)[3] While insulin is secreted into the bloodstream from the beta cells in the pancreas in response to high levels of blood sugars, glucagon is secreted from the alpha cells in the pancreas in response to low levels of blood sugar.

Glucagon pulls stored sugars out of storage, first from the liver and then from adipose or fat tissue as it converts fatty tissue back into glucose. The very presence of insulin in the bloodstream suppresses the release of glucagon, as does the ratio of carbohydrates to proteins in a meal. The greater the carbohydrate content of a meal, the more insulin will be secreted and the less glucagon will be secreted, tipping the scales in favor of fat storage through the dominating effect of insulin.[4] Conversely, the lower the carbohydrate content of the meal (or more accurately, the more balanced the meal among proteins, carbohydrates, and fats), the less insulin is secreted in favor of glucagon release.

Glucagon is stimulated by exercise[5] and a number of amino acids, but it is primarily stimulated by a diet that is fairly low in carbohydrates and a little higher in proteins and fats than many of us are accustomed to eating. In other words, by our unwitting dietary choices, we are underutilizing this "friend of the dieter" in favor of glucagon's more aggressive sister, insulin.

TAMING INSULIN'S INTENSITY

Insulin, while performing lifesaving functions like leveling out blood sugar levels, does so by increasing the risk of heart and other diseases and by contributing to obesity. The normal concentration of blood sugar is from 80 to 120 milligrams of glucose for each 100 milliliters of blood.[6]

We understand that insulin is somehow associated with diabetes and that insulin's job is to bring down excessively high levels of blood sugar. Type II diabetics have either lost the ability to secrete enough insulin to keep blood sugar levels in check or have developed a condition called insulin resistance, which essentially "locks" insulin out of target cells and keeps it circulating at high levels, a major risk factor in the development of cardiovascular and artery diseases. Insulin regulatory mechanisms break down from weak genetics, obesity, or from the overuse of blood sugar homeostatic mechanisms (eating too much sugar!). Stress also plays a role in increased insulin resistance.[7]

> *"When I get annoyed about something I go after the largest carbonated drink I can find!"*
> **MIKE**

The role insulin plays in the body, however, is much more diverse and powerful than bringing blood sugar levels under control. As one textbook terms it, "The major function of insulin is to promote storage of ingested nutrients."[8] As a storage hormone, it has an impact on virtually every tissue in the body. Insulin's primary targets are the liver, muscles, and adipose (fat) tissue. Insulin first pulls sugars out of the bloodstream and deposits them in the liver as glycogen, then in the muscle as glycogen, and finally converts it into triglycerides for storage in fat tissue. Insulin hormone "builds" fat.

Insulin increases the synthesis of several types of fat/protein and fat/sugar complexes, such as triglycerides, cholesterol, and very low density lipoproteins (VLDL), which aid in the building of muscle tissue and deliver glucose to those muscle cells for energy. LPL (lipoprotein lipase) is an enzyme that actually pulls triglycerides into fat cells for storage; insulin increases both the production and the action of LPL and inhibits those same fat cells from converting back into blood glucose.[9]

Just keep two facts in mind as we continue this discussion: *Insulin promotes fat storage, and excess carbohydrates stimulate insulin.*

LETTING INSULIN GET THE UPPER HAND

Let's revisit the high-carb menu as it relates to insulin/glucagon balance. Those healthy-looking menus from the diets espoused by Barnard, McDougall, and the Diamonds stoke your furnace with grains, fruits, and vegetables but are deficient in two macronutrients—protein and fat (essential fatty acids)—that help slow down the release of sugars into the bloodstream.

When protein and fat accompany carbohydrates into the stomach, digestion is slowed, allowing the release of sugars into the bloodstream in a time-release manner. In other words, the sugars are not just dumped into the bloodstream, which would generate a gush of insulin; they are slowly released into the bloodstream, providing a steadier stream of glucose to the brain and peripheral tissues. Because the energy is used immediately, insulin is not needed to store the excess.

When a meal doesn't contain an adequate amount of protein and fat to balance the carbohydrates, sugars are both digested quickly and released quickly into the bloodstream. Insulin pours from the pancreas in a desperate attempt to stabilize the critical level of blood sugar, and many of those carbohydrate calories will be stored as fat.

Why, then, doesn't everyone who eats a high carbohydrate diet get fat? Dr. Barry Sears, author of *Enter the Zone,* wrote about the role genetics plays in insulin/glucagon balance.

> People's genetic insulin responses to carbohydrates are diverse. In about 25 percent of a normal population, insulin response to carbohydrates is very blunted. When these lucky people eat excess carbohydrates, their insulin levels don't rapidly surge upward. They can consume large amounts of carbohydrates and not get hungry or fat. (These people often do very well on high-carbohydrate diets, so the dietary establishment elevates them to iconlike status to demonstrate the moral superiority of such a diet. Heck, these people just had a lucky draw in the genetic lottery.)
>
> On the other hand, 25 percent of an otherwise normal population has an unlucky genetic draw that dictates an extremely elevated insulin response to carbohydrates. These people simply have to look at a carbohydrate and they begin gaining fat.
>
> Between these two extremes lies the other 50 percent of the American population. These people respond normally to carbohydrates, which means that if they eat too much carbohydrate they'll have an elevated insulin response—not as elevated as the unluckiest 25 percent, but still elevated enough to do all the damage described above. These people will always fail on a high-carbohydrate diet. They're accused of being weak-willed gluttons who can't control themselves, when in fact they were just born with unfortunate genes.[10]

Yes, some people will do well on high carbohydrate diets such as those found in the Diamonds' book, *Fit for Life*, or the McDougall Plan. These people can eat carbohydrates willy-nilly and never suffer the unpleasant consequences of excess carbs like the rest of us. And sometimes, they do radiate a certain moral superiority about it.

The rest of us, for reasons as diverse as our lifestyles or the way our bodies are made, aren't so lucky. When we eat a diet high in carbohydrates, our bodies are thrown into hormonal imbalance and we're sensitive to even the good carbohydrates found in fruits, vegetables, and grains.

For example, Samantha commented that she notices an immediate insulin reaction when she eats rice cakes. Judy said, "I never realized how sweet vegetables are!" Please notice that rice cakes and vegetables are not "bad foods." They are terrific foods, and your body will love them *if* you eat them in balance with other foods to control the release of insulin.

If it's difficult to believe that a grain-and-vegetable-based diet will put on excess fat pounds, visit your local beef farmer and ask him how he prepares his beef for butchering. He fattens it up for market by "graining" it. He feeds the cattle extra grain to marbleize the meat—to add fat to the muscle tissue.

In that sense, we aren't any different from beef cattle. If we want to fatten ourselves up, we can "grain" ourselves and pack on the pounds, which is exactly what many of us have been doing for years in the form of whole-grain breads, spaghetti, and cereals.

insulin resistance

Insulin resistance can also contribute to weight gain. Insulin resistance is a condition in which receptor sites on the individual cell walls have lost the ability to receive insulin (and the attached sugars) through the cell wall where it can be used properly. The result is increased levels of insulin circulating throughout the blood accompanied by symptoms of low insulin levels. Essentially, insulin is locked out of the cells. Often, the resistance cannot be overcome by replacing the hormone[11] and is a significant issue with many obese people.

One of the most common causes of insulin resistance is obesity itself. As fat in the body accumulates, glucose tolerance diminishes. As the cells become increasingly impervious to the effects of insulin, the whole cycle of pulling glucose into the liver and muscle cells to be burned as energy gets disrupted. In the process, thyroid function is pulled down. As a matter of fact, the whole system of burning food for energy (thus reducing the tendency to store it for future use in BAT cells) shuts down, and the weight just piles on, unimpeded by glucagon or other weight-favoring hormones.[12]

For other people, the overconsumption of processed fats such as margarine, polyunsaturated oil, and other oils has contributed to insulin resistance.[13] In a letter to the editor in *The Townsend Letter for Doctors,* Jeffrey Moss, D.D.S., wrote:

> One of the most intriguing and least-known aspects of the insulin model of disease is that it also incorporates ingestion of certain types of fat, specifically, saturated fat, linoleic acid, long chain fatty acids (EPA, EFA, and arachidonic acid), and trans fats. This connection particularly fascinates me because even though we have talked about the dangers and benefits of the above fats, we have never before, as far as I know, been readily able to place these fats into a unified concept of disease that also includes subjects as diverse as ingestion of fruit, physical activity, and stress. . . . [One researcher] presents compelling evidence that not only does saturated fat raise insulin resistance, but

linoleic acid and trans fats do the same. Since the Western diet has seen a tremendous increase in the intake of linoleic acid and trans fat due to indiscriminate use of vegetable oils and margarines, this finding is particularly significant.[13]

Did you catch the meaning of what Moss is saying? Those of us who have stripped our cupboards bare of butter in favor of "heart healthy" margarine and corn oil are doing it all wrong! The "trans" fats to which Moss is referring are the artificially saturated fats like margarine and shortening and all foods that contain these fats. Corn and other vegetable oils (except for olive oil and other select vegetable oils) are implicated here as well. These foods are creating a problem with insulin resistance that keeps us heavy and just a little unbalanced in our blood sugar.

Aside from obesity or eating too much of the wrong kinds of fats, there is another cause of insulin resistance. We can be born with enzyme defects that prevent insulin from being taken up and used by the cells. But let's be honest about it: Most of the time we do it to ourselves! A high-carbohydrate diet wears out the insulin-binding capacity of the cell, as can obesity or muscle inactivity. In other words, sitting around all day eating bonbons and gaining a few extra pounds wears out your body's ability to use insulin effectively and keep circulating insulin levels down so that you're not so prone to store those excess carbs as body fat.[14]

THE ROLE OF MINERALS IN BALANCING BLOOD SUGAR

If you are deficient in several important blood sugar regulating minerals, your body just can't get the job done efficiently for you. There are several minerals involved in increasing insulin sensitivity, balancing insulin and glucagon, and reducing insulin re-sistance. The first of these minerals is *chromium.*

> *"I had hopes, but was not totally convinced that at age sixty-three I could lose my unwanted weight. In five months I lost thirty pounds and my blood pressure and cholesterol had dropped."*
>
> P.E.

Chromium is a trace mineral that was discovered in 1797 by a French chemist, but its biological significance was not deter-mined until the late fifties when researchers learned how impor-tant this mineral is in the human body. They initially found that feeding chromium to rats corrected abnormal metabolism of sugar. Later work established that chromium is a cofactor with insulin and is essential for normal glucose utilization, for growth and longevity.[15]

Hand in hand with nicotinic acid (niacin) and glutathione (a metabolic derivative of the amino acid glutamine), chromium forms a complex called the glucose tolerance factor, which is critically involved in the function of insulin. Chromium is also required for normal fat and carbohydrate metabolism.

Here we run into a problem with our twentieth-century food supply. One textbook captured the problem succinctly:

> If indeed chromium is essential to the normal metabolism
> of glucose, this mineral may illustrate a nutritional irony of
> modern times. Its distribution in foods is largely unknown,
> but it is recognized that refining removes most of all the

chromium in the typical diet. At the same time, people in Western nations are probably increasing their need for chromium by consuming large amounts of sugars and other refined carbohydrate-containing foods. The net result could be marginal chromium deficiency that catapults sensitive adults into mature-onset diabetes.[16]

The problem is not that food doesn't contain adequate amounts of chromium; the problem is that we've refined it out of our naturally produced food, or we've chosen not to eat the foods that contain it—foods like brewer's yeast, oysters, liver, and potatoes. Other foods, such as seafoods, poultry, beef, and some grains, also contain trace amounts, but the average American only gets about 33 micrograms per day in his diet, whereas we need at least 200 micrograms. Strenuous exercise and physical trauma also increases urinary excretion of chromium.[17]

There are a number of chromium deficiency symptoms, including

Elevated blood sugar	Impaired growth
Impaired glucose tolerance (inability of the cells to pick up and use blood sugar)	Decreased fertility and sperm count
	Aortic plaques
Elevated insulin levels	Elevated cholesterol levels
Glycosuria (blood sugar spilling into the urine)	Decreased longevity

We know that in the presence of high amounts of glucose in the blood, chromium is swept out of the bloodstream. Some is excreted in the urine and some simply disappears. One author wrote that "the more insulin we secrete to process sugars from a meal, the more chromium we use and lose. And once used, the mineral is discarded like a wet paper towel. As might be expected, when there's not enough chromium available, the body simply pumps out more insulin."[18] We've seen the results of more insulin as fat deposited on our hips and thighs!

Nearly all of us can benefit from supplemental chromium, but particularly those of us who have trouble controlling both our weight and our blood sugar. As a clinical nutritionist, I have recommended chromium supplementation to a number of my overweight and sugar-craving clients who notice an immediate diminishment of cravings for sweets. A side benefit of chromium may be increased ability to form lean muscle tissue, thus increasing the overall metabolic activity of the body.

Another mineral that is absolutely critical for blood sugar regulation and insulin activity is the little known mineral *manganese* (not to be confused with magnesium, another essential mineral). Manganese is a component of numerous enzymes, but it is also associated with sugar and fat metabolism. One study reported that "manganese-deficient rats exhibited reduced insulin activity, impaired glucose transport, as well as lowered insulin-stimulated glucose oxidation and conversion to triglycerides in adipose cells.[19]

While we don't need very much manganese (about 2.5 milligrams a day), we do need it very badly, and deficiencies lead to lessened insulin sensitivity in fat tissue and a decreased ability

> "When I started I was 198
> lbs. Now, I am 168 lbs and
> still losing weight."
> **JORDAN**

to transport glucose through the blood and metabolize it for energy.[20] Deficiency symptoms for manganese include impaired glucose tolerance (or the inability to regulate blood sugar levels), reduced HDL and total serum cholesterol, certain forms of mental illness like schizophrenia (other minerals may be implicated in schizophrenia as well), disc and cartilage problems, reduced brain function, middle-ear imbalances, birth defects, reduced fertility, and growth retardation.[21] Some studies have also shown that manganese deficiency can even cause an inability in mothers to bond with their newborn babies.

Vanadium, named after the Scandinavian goddess of beauty, youth, and luster,[22] has just recently come to the forefront of nutritional studies, particularly as it relates to insulin activity. Vanadium not only improves the metabolism of fats,[23] but according to one author,

> Vanadium was already a medically recommended treatment for diabetes and some forms of fatigue in the late nineteenth century in the English-speaking world. The 1932 edition of *Dorland's Medical Dictionary* listed vanadium as a treatment for diabetes and neurasthenia (mental and physical fatigue or weakness). Although not as successful as injected insulin for the treatment of extreme cases of diabetes (which is the reason it originally disappeared from medical usage) vanadium in the form of vanadyl sulfate (its biologically active form) can mimic many of the activities of insulin. In this respect, vanadyl sulfate is even more impressive than is chromium. Chromium potentiates the body's insulin, but the vanadyl form of vanadium itself is biologically active even in the absence of insulin. It significantly increases liver glycogen (stored glucose) and it improves the uptake of glucose by muscle tissues. These actions help to spare lean tissue dur-

ing dieting and to improve athletic performance by lessen-
ing fatigue and by reducing the breakdown of muscle protein for energy. . . . Nevertheless, it also acts to inhibit the
storage of excess calories from carbohydrates as fat apparently by stabilizing the body's production of insulin.[24]

Magnesium is another major mineral often overshadowed by
its complementary yet oppositional mineral—calcium. Magnesium is critically important for energy production on a cellular
level and is a major component of bone structure. Magnesium is
used to synthesize the very code of life, DNA and RNA, and
functions in nerve transmission throughout the brain and body.

Magnesium is part of many enzyme systems throughout the
body. Both magnesium and zinc are found in high concentrations
in the hippocampus (the area of the brain used for the integration
of thoughts, memory, and emotion).[25] Magnesium also helps
maintain tissue sensitivity to insulin; that is, adequate amounts
of magnesium may help prevent insulin resistance.[26] Magnesium
helps control glucose metabolism and participates in the regulation of insulin.[27]

These facts become even more important when we look at a
list of magnesium deficiency symptoms. This is where science
becomes very personal! Check this list to see how many of these
symptoms sound familiar to your body.

If you experience four, five, or more of these symptoms on a
regular basis, you may benefit from supplemental magnesium.

Some nutritionists have estimated that for many reasons up
to 65 percent of the American population is deficient in this important mineral. First, magnesium is routinely stripped out of the
food supply, but more important, we choose not to eat foods that
are potentially rich in magnesium, such as green leafy vegetables, nuts, soybeans, and crustacean seafoods—oysters and

are you deficient in zinc?

Here are some typical symptoms of zinc deficiency:

White spots on the fingernails

Cravings for carbohydrates, particularly wheat products

Lowered immune function

Dry skin or other skin problems

Impaired wound healing

Loss of the sense of taste and smell

Reduced appetite or eating disorders (anorexia, bulimia)

Loss of the desire to eat protein foods or loss of the ability to digest protein

Depression

Aggressive, hostile feelings

Fatigue

Inability to concentrate, focus, or other "mental" symptoms

Frequent frontal headaches

crabs. Because stress, sugars, and a diet high in calcium rob the body of what little magnesium it receives from food, deficiencies may be magnified many times over.

Be sure to check your magnesium intake if, in an attempt to avoid osteoporosis or other degenerative conditions, you use calcium supplements or dairy products. Excessive calcium in relation to magnesium contributes to magnesium deficiency.

In previous chapters we've talked about the importance of *zinc* in the human diet. Zinc is used in over two hundred enzyme systems in the brain alone, but it is also a critical force in the

are you magnesium deficient?

Short-term memory loss

Emotional ups and downs

Easily depressed or discouraged

Easily angered

Unfounded fears and apprehensions

Wakefulness in the middle of the night and inability to
    get back to sleep

Panic and anxiety attacks

Constipation

Cravings for chocolate and/or sweets

Muscle tremors and twitches

Muscle cramps

Palpitations of the heart

Sensitivity to loud noises

High blood pressure

Increased perspiration

regulation of blood sugar. Interestingly, one of the most common of the zinc deficiencies is a craving for carbohydrates, especially a craving for wheat-based products. Zinc-deficient people typically crave breads, pastries, and pastas.

When it comes to maintaining normal weight, you don't want to shortchange yourself on this nutrient. Zinc is used along with vanadium to potentiate insulin's ability to regulate blood sugar.

If you experience three or more of these symptoms on a regular basis you may benefit from supplemental zinc.

the glycemic index

One concept useful in weight management is the glycemic index, a rough system for rating how quickly sugars from different foods are absorbed into the bloodstream, affecting a subsequent rise in blood sugar. Dr. Richard Podell, M.D., author of *The G-Index Diet: The Missing Link That Makes Permanent Weight Loss Possible,* explains it like this:

> Foods that have a *low* Glycemic Index (GI) are best for dieters because they promote a slow, moderate rise in blood sugar and insulin after a meal—factors that help keep hunger in check. These same factors also encourage the body to dissolve body fat by converting it into energy.
>
> In contrast, *high* GI foods cause sudden, unstable swings in blood sugar, first with very high sugar and insulin surges, then with a crash of the sugar toward excessively low levels. The end result is increased appetite and irritability—and a great tendency to convert food calories into body fat.
>
> In short, the goal of the dieter is to build a food plan around *low* Glycemic Index foods. This way, hunger is minimized, and there is less tendency to overeat. Consequently, the dieter can continue to lose weight—or to maintain an ideal weight once the excess pounds have been lost.[28]

There are three primary factors that determine the glycemic index of a food: the fiber content, the structure of the sugar (simple or complex), and the fat content.

Glucose, a simple sugar, is absorbed very quickly into the bloodstream because of its chemical structure and is found predominately in grains (pasta, bread, and cereals), starches, and many vegetables. Fructose has to be converted to glucose in the liver and enters the bloodstream more slowly. Fructose is naturally found in most fruits but can be synthesized from corn. (Remember that corn is high on our list of allergenic foods.) Foods that are high in fiber will go into the bloodstream more slowly, which is why juicing will not be a good idea if your blood sugar is unstable or if you have a weight problem.

When you begin putting your meal plan together based on the information to follow, you will want to strictly limit foods that are high on the glycemic index (foods that cause blood sugar levels to soar) and enjoy foods that are low on the Glycemic Index to encourage the secretion of glucagon.

A general list of high-glycemic foods includes:

All grains (including whole wheat and rice products)

Most processed foods, particularly those with added sugars

Starchy foods like potatoes, carrots, and corn

Fruit, particularly grapes, oranges, and other high-sugar fruits

As you will find from our sample menus in chapter 8, you may indulge in these high-glycemic foods occasionally *if* you carefully balance them with proteins and fats to slow down the release of sugars into the bloodstream. Until you have worked with the program for a while and are familiar with it, I strongly suggest you avoid the use of all these foods. If you do, you will feel better, it will be easier to keep your blood sugar under control, and your weight will drop more quickly.

the bottom line

Let's go back and recapture the principles outlined in this chapter. If it seems too technical, too complicated, too *medical-ese*, take a little extra time with it because the issues are so important. If you can firmly grasp the concept that excessive carbohydrates increase blood levels of insulin, that insulin is a storage hormone that converts those carbohydrates into stored body fat, and that the only way to control insulin is through controlling the amount of carbohydrates you eat at every meal, you can start to understand why your weight struggle started in the first place. You can see for the first time in your overweight life that obesity is not primarily (or even secondarily) a matter of calorie counting or cutting fat out of your diet. It is not just a matter of self-control. And for most readers, it is not even a matter of genetics or thyroid or brown fat or allergies.

Losing excess fat is a matter of controlling blood sugars. By controlling blood sugars, you control the storage of fat. The equation is simple: Excessive Carbohydrates = Fat Tissue. That's it! That's the bottom line!

If you're reading this book, you're probably either in the unlucky lower 25 percent of the population who respond violently to surges of excess carbohydrates in the diet (I'm in the lower end of the gene pool), or you may be in the 50 percent in the middle who respond well to the type of diet we advocate, which is substantially different from the high-carbohydrate/low-fat diets so popular in the press and the rest of our culture.

You're going to have to find your way out of the muddle of information about so-called weight-loss programs and start looking at the *real* reason you struggle with weight. Chances are you overrespond to carbohydrates and are putting on weight because of high insulin levels circulating in your blood. An occasional indulgence in high-carbohydrate foods will not substantially alter how your body turns those carbohydrates into fat; but the continual, deliberate overconsumption of large amounts of carbohydrates will.

It's common knowledge in both the research and clinical worlds that a balanced diet will essentially shut down an excessive production of insulin and allow glucagon full access to your vast stores of energy. This knowledge just hasn't reached mainstream America yet. Frankly, there isn't a lot of excitement about dietary balance. Crazy schemes that involve grapefruit, fiber, or herbal stimulants get a lot more press.

Winning the weight game involves balancing your diet by using the macronutrients called protein, fat, and carbohydrates to stimulate the release of glucagon. No fancy programs or expensive clinics. No pills to swallow and no creams to rub on your thighs. You don't need to buy running shoes or abdominal reducers (although moderate exercise does help stimulate glucagon). You can work the concepts of this book into your family meals at home, your favorite restaurant dining, your business lunches, and when you eat at a friend's house.

It's time for you to start making good use of all those calories you've been saving, and believe me, you have more than enough stored calories! The average 150-pound person stores over

> *"It is now second nature to me to make food selections that agree with my body's metabolism. . . . It is a lifestyle change that can and will make you fat-free for life!"*
> **JORDAN**

100,000 calories in the form of triglycerides just waiting for the opportunity to be used. And because balancing insulin and glucagon is the healthiest, most balanced way to use those calories for energy, your body will love you for it.

We've spent a lot of time discussing complex hormonal issues. Now it's time to lay it all aside and learn what I mean when I say "balanced diet." To hear some people tell it, a balanced diet is a cup of coffee and a bagel (something wet and something dry!), a bowl of ice cream and a chocolate chip cookie (something white and something brown!), or a plate of pasta and a salad (something big and something small!). When I talk about dietary balance, I'm talking about something a little more complex, a little more sensible, and a *lot* healthier! I'm talking about a diet that will bring your body back into homeostasis and let the pounds melt away like butter on a hot summer day.

The
Good
News

7

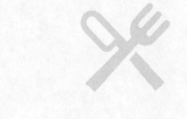

You've heard the depressing story of why all those diets you've tried over the past twenty years have failed. You've seen why your own body chemistry is fighting you. Now it's time to put the depressing news aside and look at some good news. Even though your body is uncooperative and you've tried and failed miserably in the past, you can finally succeed—permanently. It may not even be difficult for you; all you have to do is learn how to do it, and then do it!

controlled, not cured

Before you start on your own personal weight-loss program, using my guidelines, you must accept one fact: Your weight problem is permanent. I've said it before, but I need to say it again so you don't make the mistake of taking on this project as a "summer diet" or a "three-month plan" or to diet just until you get your weight down to where you want it. To really succeed in weight management over the long term, you will never again be able to look at food as casually as you have until this point. Now you must view yourself just as though you were an alcoholic.

Before an alcoholic can recover, he must acknowledge: "I am an alcoholic." He has to recognize the fact that he will remain an alcoholic throughout his lifetime, even if he never touches another drop of alcohol. He is permanently alcoholic.

You are permanently overweight. Remember that, because if you follow my program for a few months, drop your excess weight, and resume your old eating patterns, you will regain every pound of fat you lost, plus several more. You've seen why this happened in the past, and it *will* happen again. Your old weight will return with a vengeance, and you'll feel just as bad as you did before. You can NEVER resume your old way of eating without suffering the consequences. In a very tangible sense, you have a physical disability that you cannot cure; you can only control it. You have a *permanent* weight problem!

In those two words, "control it," you can literally set yourself free, because even though you can't cure your obesity, you need never be fat again! Some of you are going to find it difficult to set aside some foods you love dearly in exchange for foods that don't offer as much sensuous gratification. But stay with me, because I offer you the tools to permanently change how much you weigh, even if I can't "cure" your weight problem. I offer you the tools to reshape the health of your body!

Throughout this book I have stressed the principle of dietary balance. I'm not advocating some faddish, off-the-wall diet plan that sets you up for failure at the end of the program. I'm teaching you the secret of permanent weight control, which is the balance of dietary proteins, fats, and carbohydrates at every meal, every time you put food in your mouth. I want dietary balance to become second nature to you so that whenever and wherever you eat, you'll automatically put these principles to work for you.

the three macronutrients

PROTEIN

Because protein is the most complicated food to add to the high-carbohydrate diets we're used to, we'll start by discussing the role of protein and protein requirements in the body and how to meet those requirements—meal by meal. Once you begin to understand just how important proteins are, it will be easier to include them in your diet.

When we discuss the need for protein in the body, we're really talking about the end result of protein digestion—amino acids—because intact protein is unusable to the body. When you think of protein, think of a pearl necklace—tiny iridescent beads strung together on a cord that binds them together in the pattern designed by the artist. Protein is a gestalt of amino acids, minerals, and vitamins strung together in precise configuration on a peptide bond. Some proteins are simple, containing only a few dozen amino acids. Others are amazingly complicated with literally hundreds of amino acids, precisely ordered and twisted into a shape that conforms to the design laid down by DNA.

When a protein food reaches the stomach, powerful enzymes uncoil each of the molecules, then begin to break the peptide bonds apart, making smaller and smaller protein chains that are finally cleaved into individual amino acids as they pass through the corridor of the small intestine. These amino acids are welcomed through the intestinal lining into the bloodstream where they are used to reconfigure over 300,000 different protein molecules.

> *"I am grateful to Carol for this weight-loss program. It's an absolute blessing to me."*
> **SARAH**

To give you an idea of the range of functions these proteins perform, consider this short list of protein bodies: immune cells; nerve tissue; muscle tissue; visceral tissue such as the stomach, liver, pancreas, esophagus; enzymes; hormones; neurotransmitters; and iron-binding molecules. The list is much longer, but just keep in mind that every functioning structure in the body is made up of protein, along with cofactors of minerals and vitamins.

It's easy to see how important it is to get enough protein in the diet, but beyond total protein consumption, how critically important that we receive all eight to ten essential amino acids daily. If even *one* amino acid is in short supply, some structure will not be synthesized, some function will not be performed. Over time, poor health will result.

How much protein do you need? The average woman requires about forty-five to seventy-five grams of protein a day just to build these 300,000 body structures. The average man requires from fifty-five to eighty-five grams of protein a day for the same reason. Many nutritionists use this simple formula to determine a person's individual need for protein: Divide your weight by 2.2. This is your weight in kilograms. Multiply your kilogram weight by 0.8. This is your base protein requirement.

> Do you have trouble understanding how much real food equals a gram or more of protein? Animal proteins (seafood, poultry, veal) contain roughly 9 grams of protein per ounce. The average egg contains 6.2 grams of protein. From there, it's easy to do the mathematics to achieve your protein goal!

There are a number of conditions that may change this protein requirement. For example, both men and women under stress require slightly more protein by increasing the requirement and activity of certain hormones (adrenal hormones, for example) and by increasing the metabolic rate of the body. Long-term stress is associated with conversion of protein to carbohydrate and fat, resulting in weight gain and elevation in serum fats.[1]

The term *nitrogen balance* refers to the balance between protein coming into the body through diet or being recycled after its initial use, and the demands of the body. When we refer to "negative nitrogen balance," it simply means that we're using or burning more protein than is being replaced. If negative nitrogen balance continues for a long period of time, eventually the body starts breaking down muscle and other lean tissue to provide for other more critical needs like hormones, enzymes, and neurotransmitters.

Unrelenting stress leads to a negative nitrogen balance that can only be balanced by either relieving the stress or increasing the amount of usable protein. If you are dogged by unrelenting stress that you can't resolve right now, add another five, even *ten*, grams of protein to your diet. Men under stress require more protein, but women particularly need to be aware of their protein intake during times of physical or emotional stress. Pregnancy and lactation impose an even greater need for protein. This is not the time to go on a protein-restricted diet!

If you are physically very active, you will need a few more grams of protein each day. If you enjoy a light workout several times a week, you may need to add about five grams. On the other hand, if your job is physically demanding and after work you enjoy stopping by the gym for a couple of hours to pump iron, you may need to add ten or more grams of additional protein. If your body just "runs fast" (fast metabolism), you may feel free to be more generous in your protein intake.

> *"All attempts in the past to lose weight left me feeling unacceptable and a failure."*
> SARAH

It's tempting to cite a specific formula for determining your exact protein requirement and from that calculate the amount of carbohydrate you need, and then determine your fat allowance for the day. This brings the science of endocrine balance into a precision that is extremely valuable. The problem with this type of precision is the difficulty you will have in calculating the amount and type of food you need divided into protein/carbohydrate/fat units. This is where virtually every sensible weight-loss program fails; it's just too difficult to figure out and to plan your meals.

As a nutritionist who works with *real people*, I've found it more useful to give my clients a rough idea of their protein requirements (based on the information given above) and then allow their bodies to fine-tune it for them.

I encourage you to listen to your body. Eat *slowly* just until you are satisfied, then stop! You'll be amazed how easily your body communicates how much food it needs for your optimum health and vitality.

CARBOHYDRATES

After reading chapter 6 on maintaining your insulin balance, you may be thinking you should avoid carbohydrates at all cost since they can so easily increase insulin secretion, which packs on additional pounds of fat weight. Carbohydrates, however, are an essential part of the diet. As long as you enjoy them in balance with protein and fats, they will do just the job they were originally intended to do—provide energy to the body.

Carbohydrates, or sugars, are the fuels your body burns in each of its three trillion-plus cells to provide energy. The brain "runs" on carbohydrates (or sugars). Carbohydrates are the quickest, most readily available source of energy, and when carbohydrates are no longer available, the body burns fat, then protein. If carbohydrates are underprovided, the body is often forced to cannibalize lean body tissue to provide fuel. So it's important to eat enough carbohydrates to satisfy the body's energy requirement each day.

Select carbohydrates that are low on the glycemic index (see chapter 6 for this information) and avoid foods that precipitously increase blood sugar. You would do well to virtually eliminate all starchy foods, such as potatoes, yams, carrots, corn, grain products, and rice that so easily increase blood sugar. Feel free to indulge in as many "greens" as you wish. Green foods are free foods!

The more scientific way to calculate your carbohydrate needs is to multiply the amount of protein you require by 1.3. Use this chart as a handy guide:

Protein:	Carbohydrate:
55 g.	71.5 g.
65 g.	84.5 g.
75 g.	97.5 g.
85 g.	110.5 g.
95 g.	123.5 g.

The problem most people have with this chart is learning what constitutes 71.5 grams of carbohydrates, or 65 grams of protein. Here are a couple of tools to put this information in a format you can use to prepare your meals.

Most animal-based proteins (seafood, poultry, veal, lamb, beef) contain about 9 grams of protein per ounce. If you require 65 grams of protein per day, plan to use about 7 1/2 ounces of seafood, poultry, or other protein per day, divided between breakfast, lunch, and dinner.

By the way, the premise of this book does not allow for a totally vegetarian lifestyle. Those who eat eggs and dairy products as part of the protein source can easily become allergic to these foods through overconsumption, and soy products will put weight on a person who is either estrogen sensitive or for whom soy pulls down the activity of the thyroid gland.

Another way to measure the amount of protein you will need at each meal is to use the palm of your hand. Plan to eat a protein portion about the size of the palm of your hand. Carbohydrates can fill up the rest of the plate, as long as you are *not* using any starchy vegetables, sweetened beverages, or fruit.

Remember this simple rule: You must include a protein portion *with each meal* if you wish to slow down the entry of sugars into your bloodstream and encourage your pancreas to secrete glucagon instead of insulin. Insulin = Fat! No more high-carb meals or snacks!

If you have indulged freely in carbohydrates (either the "good carbs" or the "bad" carbs), you are going to find this approach a little difficult to swallow, especially if you've been working with the vegetable/grain base type of diet. I'm going to offer you a little grace, a little leeway in starting your program, because for you this may be an enormous change in lifestyle.

When I counsel clients using this prototype, I watch their faces while I'm unrolling the plan. If they pale, if their expression goes blank, or they stand up and say, "I can't do this! I'm outta here!" I change my approach! After all, I want them to succeed, not secede!

I encourage you to take one meal at a time (dinner, for example) and work on balancing that one meal until you are totally comfortable with the plan. This may take just a few days; it may take a few weeks. But in that one meal, make sure the proteins and carbohydrates are balanced so carefully that you begin to feel a difference. You may even start to lose a little weight!

*The host of the party was
serving fresh-sliced
watermelon. "That's okay.
That's okay," I said. But
after a while it just hit me. I
saw those slices cut into
fourths, and I said, "Just the
heart." I tried to find the
biggest piece, took it, and
stood there and ate the heart.
I just let the juice run down
my chin and over my hand,
and I said, "I'm going to
cherish this moment."*

J.H.

When you are totally comfortable with dinner, do lunch. Either enjoy leftovers from the evening meal or use some of the lunch suggestions in the recipe section of this book (Appendix A). Work with both lunch and dinner for a few weeks until this new way of eating is ingrained into your psyche. Before you know it, eating a balanced meal will seem like second nature to you.

And by the way, don't worry if you "blow it" occasionally. We all do. Just start over again at the next meal and carry on. Your body is a wonderful organism; it has grace built into it. It can handle the occasional nutritional disaster. Just make sure you get back on track as soon as possible and make those occasional "slips" as infrequently as possible. And if you're tempted to blow it big time, read my "cheat story" on p. 232 for information on how to cheat appropriately so that you don't suffer undue consequences. The point is to make a permanent lifestyle change, even if you occasionally eat the old way.

FAT

For the past few decades, we've been bombarded with the message "Fat is *bad* food!" Every women's magazine, every sports magazine, every men's magazine, every health magazine includes at least one article or advertisement about how the consumption of fat will subtract years from your life by causing degenerative disease, including heart disease, cancer, stroke, diabetes. To listen to the experts, you would think fat isn't an essential part of the human diet.

We've already learned that it's no accident that nature distributed fat abundantly throughout the food chain. Fat is an extremely beneficial food. For example, fat is used to build hormones, some of which regulate blood pressure, heart rate, vascular dilation, blood clotting, immune response, and the central nervous system. Fat makes up a substantial part of the cell membrane of over three trillion cells, making the cell wall permeable so that nutrients can get into the cell and waste materials can be excreted from the cell, and rigid so that the shape holds firm against the pressure of the surrounding environment. Along with protein, fat acts as a receptor on the cell wall to invite nutrients and hormones into the cell.

Fat keeps the skin soft and supple and helps to avoid premature wrinkling of the skin. Fat is an excellent energy source, particularly for the heart. And fat keeps the metabolism running fast!

We need fat in our diets. The problem comes when we eat far too much of the wrong types of fats.

An important rule of thumb I personally follow is that I never eat anything that has been put together in a chemist's lab, including new food artifacts like the "fat substitute" Olestra. These substances are toxic. They do not build the type of long-term, vibrant health I want for my body. They do not perform all those important functions listed above. On top of that, they taste bad!

what about olestra?

The term *fat substitute* is misleading because there is no biological substitute for dietary fat. The body can't replace its need for essential fats with a synthetic material. According to the Physicians' Committee for Responsible Medicine (PCRM), Olestra is bad news for everyone, including dieters.

A recent press release from PCRM stated:

> Proctor & Gamble's own documents affirm that Olestra acts as a "vitamin vacuum" that pulls fat-soluble vitamins (vitamins A, D, E, and K) from the body, along with beta-carotene and dozens of other vital cancer-fighting nutrients. Proctor & Gamble has proposed counteracting the "vitamin vacuum" effect by fortifying Olestra with vitamins, yet it has no way to determine the full range of vitamins and other compounds Olestra removes.[2]

I'm not sure what good it would do to fortify Olestra-containing foods with fat-soluble vitamins since it removes those same nutrients from the body. But because Americans are already seriously deficient in essential fatty acids and numerous other nutrients, substituting Olestra for healthy fats is not a good idea. And the side effects of Olestra use have included abdominal cramping and pain, diarrhea, and other digestive upsets, which tells us the body is not impressed with the newest food-technology product to hit the market!

Frito-Lay currently has exclusive rights to use Olestra. Frito-Lay enjoys a market share of more than 50 percent of the $15 billion snack food industry.[3]

As you read in chapter 2, the types of fats you want to include in your diet are the raw, unprocessed vegetable oils like extra-virgin olive oil, avocado oil, and the oils from nuts and seeds. You need to include the fats found in fatty fish like mackerel, salmon, and halibut. These oils are extremely beneficial in protecting the heart and nourishing the nervous system. I encourage all my clients to include at least two to four tablespoons of raw oils in their diets each day by making salad dressings from olive oil, by using flaxseed oil in their morning protein drink, and by eating vegetables that are rich in essential fats (avocados and nuts and seeds, such as sesame, almond, and other nut products). Flaxseed oil is a nutritious oil from flax that can be purchased from your local health food store. Be sure to keep it refrigerated. It oxidizes rapidly if not preserved carefully.

You will need to include about half the amount of fat as your protein requirement, gram for gram. For example, if you require fifty-five grams of protein per day, you will wish to enjoy about twenty-five to thirty grams of fat. If you require seventy-five grams of protein, increase that amount to about thirty-five to forty grams of fat. Don't worry too much about the fat content of the diet. If you are eating whole, natural foods, the fat will balance itself out without your help. Just restrict yourself to the *healthy* fats described above. Potato chips, ice cream, and deep-fried chicken must *not* be included!

step-by-step weight loss

Let's review each basic concept of weight loss to make sure you are tracking with me.

Weight-Loss Principle #1. Include a good source of protein with every meal.

When planning your meal, start with the protein. Some excellent sources of protein are fish, chicken, turkey, moderate amounts of beef, tofu, and eggs. Contrary to what you may have read in other sources, each one of these foods provides a well-balanced source of amino acids. You will want to limit beef because it can be pro-inflammatory, but you may enjoy it every two weeks or so. Always try to buy organic.

Weight-Loss Principle #2. Eat a large portion of greens with both lunch and dinner.

This can take the form of a salad (see the Basic Salad recipe in Appendix A) or lightly steamed greens like beans or broccoli. You may also include other vegetables, such as cauliflower, tomatoes, cucumbers, onions, jicama, and others. There are over one hundred varieties of vegetables on the American market. Learn to enjoy them. Season with lots of herbs, garlic, or a little butter. Be creative!

Weight-Loss Principle #3. Strictly limit foods that are high in carbohydrates.

Limit foods like rice, potatoes, sweet potatoes, corn, and most of all, grains. Especially be careful to avoid all bread and pasta products. I know of no surer way to start dropping excess weight than by eliminating all wheat products from your diet!

Refer back to the Glycemic Index in chapter 6 and avoid foods that are high on the glycemic index. With every meal, include a protein portion along with beneficial fats to further slow the release of sugars into the bloodstream.

Weight-Loss Principle #4. Exercise moderately every day.

Check with your physician before embarking on an exercise program, especially if you are more than twenty-five pounds overweight or you have a physical condition that must be monitored by a professional. Even if your condition is compromised by obesity or another health challenge, your doctor can put together a program that will be right for you.

Don't take lightly my injunction to exercise. If you are going to achieve weight control and maintain your overall health, you must get off the couch and get moving! Your body was meant to move, not to sit. Every part of your body will work better if you are involved in regular, sustained exercise.

> Exercise helps relieve symptoms of asthma, improves your mood, and benefits your cardiovascular system.

> Exercise lifts depression, reduces the risk of colon cancer, and helps normalize insulin levels.

> Exercise is good for your back and your bones and helps reduce the risk of osteoporosis.

> Exercise increases the production of endorphins and reduces chronic pain.

> Exercise makes you think more clearly.

> Exercise increases your metabolic rate by stimulating the activity of your thyroid gland.

> Exercise reduces stress, which reduces toxic levels of cortisone and other stress hormones.

> Exercise builds muscles, which makes your body burn calories more efficiently and reduces the risk of obesity.

> Exercise helps control diabetes and menstrual cycles.

Name one part of the body and I'll name at least one benefit that body part will receive from exercise! One physician felt so strongly about exercise that he titled one of the chapters in his book "If You Can't Walk, Crawl."[4]

We all know that exercise burns calories. Professional dieters know exactly how many calories each type of exercise will burn and how long it takes! But beyond its calorie-burning capacity, exercise helps build lean muscle tissue—the ally of the chronically obese.

Skeletal muscle makes up about 45 percent of the total body mass and is metabolically active, depending on the amount of physical activity engaged in. Energy production, therefore, is enhanced by increasing the activity and size of the muscle mass of the body, particularly the cardiac and skeletal muscles. Put simply, the more muscle you have, the more energy you burn, and the easier it is to trim your figure.

If you want to balance your energy requirements, you want to build more muscle in relation to fat. And this is the primary reason the chronically overweight person needs to exercise. Exercise increases the metabolic rate of the entire body.

I am probably the best person to discuss exercise because I loathe it. I don't like walking (it's boring), riding bikes (it's dangerous), running (it's painful), swimming (I don't know how), or aerobics (all of the above). I've never enjoyed any activity more strenuous than strolling through my flower garden or pecking away at my computer.

But when I started complaining about recurring back problems, weight gain, hormonal challenges, and numerous other "age-related" conditions, my naturopathic doctor gently started nagging me: "Started your exercise program yet? Your back will stop hurting when you start exercising. Hmmm, not exercising yet, are you?" Finally, I listened to him, got up off the chair, put an exercise video into the video machine, and started moving around a little.

> *"To my enjoyment, Carol has introduced me to a whole new way of eating that satisfies my hunger and meets my nutritional needs, with even a few goodies thrown in."*
>
> **CANDACE**

I'm not going to tell you my workout time is my favorite part of the day (I'm a truthful woman). But I will say that my back doesn't hurt anymore. I'm more flexible, I can walk up a flight of stairs without suffering cardiac arrest, and my hormones have settled down into a comfortable pattern. I'm not as stressed, and I get some of my most creative ideas on the treadmill. I'm losing that extra five pounds of fat, too.

While I don't particularly like to exercise, I *love* the way my body feels when I do it. And that is enough motivation for even this middle-aged, sedentary woman!

Weight-Loss Principle #5 Drink water!

What *is* and what *is not* water? Water is water (with a little lemon or lime juice for flavor, if desired). Water is caffeine-free herbal teas. Water is not coffee, soft drinks, or fruit juice. Water is not soup or any other beverage. Water is water. Period.

Your body is over 65 percent water. Water is just as essential to the body as food and is used for extremely critical body functions. For example, every enzymatic reaction that occurs in the body requires water. Without it, life ceases. Maintaining that 65 percent water content is so important that even if your body drops just 1 percent fluid level, dehydration sets in, and if the body becomes just 5 percent dehydrated, serious health consequences follow. You must drink water! By the time you feel thirsty, you're already 1 percent dehydrated.

You need to drink eight to ten eight-ounce glasses of water each day just to hydrate the tissues and eliminate toxic waste. Most people drink far less than that amount. It is especially critical to increase water intake during weight loss, because as the body drops its load of fat, a certain amount of toxins are released into the bloodstream and sent to the liver and kidneys. You've got to give these organs enough water to move the waste out of the body.

Weight-Loss Principle #6 Avoid all nonfoods. I know you've been taught that as long as a food is low-fat or fat-free it is healthy, but that simply isn't true! Most of the "food" on the American market is not food. Oh, it looks like food, but it doesn't fulfill any requirements of the human body. What do these nonfoods include?

> *"The luscious recipes Carol provided brought the joy back into cooking."*
> **MARY**

Nonfoods are all carbonated beverages, all canned foods, and all processed foods. Nonfoods include highly allergenic foods like dairy and wheat products, corn and corn-based products like fructose, coffee, tea, and anything with artificial flavors or preservatives. Nonfoods are rancid oils like margarine, shortening, and any food made with these unhealthy fats. Nonfoods include such common supermarket items as potato chips, corn chips, cookies, pastries, bagels, simulated fruit beverages, or anything that comes in a box, a can, or a wrapper.

Nonfoods are pseudofoods that have never been alive. Our list of nonfoods also includes all foods to which you are allergic (often the foods you love most dearly!).

Unfortunately, the average person has been brainwashed that it's okay to eat anything as long as it's low in fat or sugar. We feel virtuous when we eat foods and beverages sweetened with aspartame or munch on low-fat potato chips, crackers, cookies . . . you name it.

If you've been taught that low-fat is healthy, no matter what the food, then it's imperative that you make a shift in your thinking. I'll admit, it won't be easy to give up these favorite foods. But once you discover the "art of feeling good," you're less likely to go back to the old way of eating. If you do lapse, you probably won't stay there for long.

Once you discover the secret of balancing your body's glucagon and insulin output by balancing what goes into your mouth, you won't want to eat any other way!

carol's rules for healthy eating:

1. Never eat anything that comes with instructions.
2. Never eat anything that comes in a box, a can, or a wrapper.
3. Never eat anything white. (Potatoes are brown; rice is beige, cauliflower is cream colored, and ice cream is nasty!)
4. Never eat anything you can't spell or pronounce.
5. Never eat anything you just *can't* live without (you're probably allergic to it).

If you are going to lose weight and keep it off, you're going to have to turn your back on the American food culture and learn to eat your ancestral diet. Your grandparents enjoyed moderate amounts of protein foods, small amounts of seasonal fruits, and lots of vegetables washed down with clean water. They ate what was in season at the time, freshly harvested. Some foods, like winter squash, potatoes, carrots, and a few other fruits and vegetables that could be stored in a cellar were saved for the winter; everything else was eaten as soon as it was picked from the field or the garden.

This is the type of diet your body was designed to eat, and it will bring your waistline back under control. It may not be the most entertaining diet. It may not excite the interest of the chic crowd. It may not catch the attention of the media. But trust me, it is the diet your body was meant to eat, and your body will reward you by dropping those excess pounds and adding years of vital health to your life.

> *"Joining Carol's program is one of the best things I have ever done for myself."*
> **KAREN**

Are you ready to get started? It's time to put these principles to work for you, in the most practical sense. Theory is one thing; putting dinner on the table is another. Let's close the classroom door now and step into the kitchen.

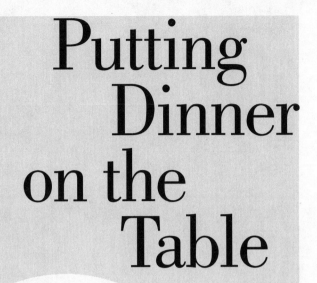

Putting Dinner on the Table

8

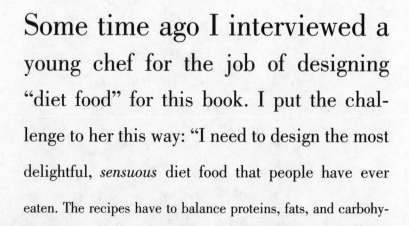

Some time ago I interviewed a young chef for the job of designing "diet food" for this book. I put the challenge to her this way: "I need to design the most delightful, *sensuous* diet food that people have ever eaten. The recipes have to balance proteins, fats, and carbohydrates in a precise 30-30-40 ratio, eliminate most common food allergens like wheat, dairy, corn, and soy, and be easy for the typical man or woman to prepare . . . and make it food that the entire family will enjoy. Oh, and it should be inexpensive."

Meg just looked at me and said, "No problem."

When Meg West and I sat down and put together this truly delightful selection of "diet food," my standards were very high because I really enjoy food! This food had to taste good!

Let me introduce you to the most delightful, *sensuous* "diet" food you've ever enjoyed. Meg designed each of these menus to fit into your busy schedule, yet tease your taste buds with combinations of foods and flavors you may never have experienced. Several of my clients have commented on how tempting each meal is and that some of their grown children are dropping by for dinner more frequently! One woman was even asked to open her own restaurant—using her "diet foods"! We think you'll be delighted as well.

Just one word of warning: The most difficult part of this menu plan may be the time factor. You need to spend a little more time in the kitchen but this doesn't have to be bad. We're so used to throwing a plate of spaghetti, a bowl of cereal, or a creamy casserole on the table that it takes some getting used to in order to plan a meal around a protein embellished with fresh vegetables and condiments of fruit. We've lost the art of culinary skills, of nourishing both soul and body in the preparation and serving of beautiful, delicious food.

The preparation of *really good food* is an important part of our culture that needs to be passed on from generation to generation. What flavors and aromas will our children remember from their childhood mealtimes? SpaghettiOs and Hamburger Helper? Boxes of KFC and containers of instant mashed potatoes topped with pseudogravy? The pizza deliveryman?

The menus that follow do require that you become reacquainted with your kitchen. You will need to spend a little more time shopping for and preparing food. You will want to stock your pantry with ingredients ahead of time so they are ready when you need them.

> *"The most important things I learned on Carol's program were how to take care of myself and live healthy for the rest of my life."*
> **KAREN**

We encourage our clients to do their grocery shopping twice a week and prepare all their vegetables before they put them away in the refrigerator. Vegetables can be washed, cut, and stored in containers in the refrigerator and last for several days if they are prepared and dried carefully. The few minutes you spend in planning and advance preparation will drastically cut down meal preparation and kitchen cleanup each evening. This is so important that we've included "Meal-in-a-Flash Prep Plans" with nearly every recipe.

As a busy wife, mother, and businesswoman, I've found that if I spend just twenty minutes in the kitchen while the kids are getting ready for school in the morning, doing these "Meal-in-a-Flash Prep Plan" ideas, I can serve dinner with minimal time in the kitchen in the evening when I'm really rushed and still caught up in the events of the day.

The menu plans that follow accomplish several goals:

1. They eliminate the foods most likely to cause allergic reactions; that is, they do not contain wheat or dairy (except for goat milk products in a few recipes), or artificial ingredients. The use of corn products is minimal.

2. They use fresh foods from the supermarket with minimal packaged foods. You will be eating *live* foods with an abundance of fresh vegetables, some fruits, and some grains. Your body will thrive on the rich variety of this diet.

3. You are allowed to eat as much of this food as you desire as long as you balance every meal carefully. In other words, each menu is carefully balanced among protein, carbohydrates, and fats. The portion size is fairly insignificant. Eat until you are satisfied. The only thing you must be careful about is not increasing just the carbohydrate portion of the meal. If you feel you need to eat a little more, increase *both* the carbohydrate and protein.

4. Each meal is designed to reduce the secretion of insulin and stimulate the release of glucagon, accomplished very simply through balancing the macronutrients. While you may change the order of the whole menu (you may eat Tuesday's menu on Wednesday, for example) you may not exchange foods within the menu for another (you may not substitute a baked potato for the salad, for example). Each menu has been put together specifically to balance out the other foods within the meal. And please remember to drink eight to ten glasses of water each day.

It can be difficult to make an abrupt change in your eating habits, so I strongly recommend that for at least the first three months (or until you are comfortable on this program) you either use a meal replacement bar or a protein drink for your breakfast meal. It can be daunting to change three meals a day, especially first thing in the morning when you're rushing out the door!

I've counseled many clients on this program and found that they were able to follow the program *if* they didn't have to think about breakfast. When I asked them to prepare three balanced meals a day, they nearly always failed. But if I recommended either a meal replacement bar or a protein drink for breakfast, they nearly always succeeded.

Most food bars are far too carbohydrate dense to qualify as an insulin-reducing meal. Even so-called high-protein bars often contain less than 15 grams of protein up against 40 or more grams of carbohydrate. And most of those carbohydrates are high Glycemic Index sugars that will jack up your blood sugar levels precipitously and stimulate an insulin response. Other bars that are well balanced between the macronutrients are so full of potential allergy-producing ingredients that I have trouble recommending them.

The only two bars I can recommend at this time are Balance bars and Ironman bars. Both of these bars (available in numerous flavors) are sold through health food stores and GNC. If you cannot obtain them locally, check Appendix C for more information.

If you don't care for a bar, you may use a protein drink for breakfast instead. Again, the issue is one of optimum balance between the macronutrients protein, carbohydrate, and fat. There are few protein powders that meet these requirements. The ones I can recommend are:

Fulfill, from Nature's Secret (mix with flax oil)

UniPro The Perfect Protein (mix with fruit and flax oil)

Nature's Life SuperPro 96 (mix with fruit and flax oil)

Nature's Plus Spirutein

These protein drinks should be available through your local health food store or GNC. If not, check Appendix C for information on how to obtain these products in your area.

There may be other protein powders that work well; simply read the ingredients carefully to make sure they contain no more than one-third more carbohydrate than protein in a serving size. For example, if one scoop of powder provides 15 grams of protein, it should contain no more than 22.5 grams of carbohydrate. If one scoop provides 20 grams of protein, it should contain no more than 30 grams of carbohydrates.

Be particularly careful to avoid artificial sweeteners, artificial coloring or flavoring agents, and preservatives. Be especially wary of the protein or meal replacement drinks promoted heavily on TV or other media; they are typically full of sweeteners (high in carbohydrates) and artificial {everything}! If you can, avoid any foods to which you may be allergic, like corn sweeteners (fructose), casein protein (protein from a dairy source—the label will read "casein . . ."), egg or dairy protein, or other foods that may be specific to your own needs.

Use the following recipe to make your breakfast drink:

1–2 *scoops of protein powder (my favorite: Fulfill by Nature's Secret) (up to 20 grams of protein per serving size)*

2 *tablespoons raw flaxseed oil*

1 *teaspoon powdered green foods (available from the health food store). I highly recommend the powdered*

greens from EarthRise, Nature's Life, Kyolic, or Magna Barley.

2–3 *cups of water (according to taste and texture)*

1 *medium-sized banana (You may wish to add a drop of vanilla for added flavor.)*

Place all ingredients in a blender container and blend thoroughly.

> Ultra Slim-Fast is the most heavily advertised meal replacement drink on the market today, but it is a nutritional disaster. Each serving contains twenty-four grams of carbohydrates (sixteen grams are in the form of sugar!) and only five grams of protein: a balance that is sure to send blood sugar levels soaring and insulin racing out of control. The number-one ingredient on the label is sugar, followed closely by cocoa. Highly allergenic foods like milk and whey are added, along with artificial flavors, artificial coloring agents, and aspartame. Aspartame has generated more letters of complaint to the FDA for side effects than any other product in the American supermarket. Is this the type of product you want to be putting into your body? I don't think so!

Now that breakfast has been taken care of, what will you eat for lunch and dinner? Pretend that you're sitting in your favorite gourmet restaurant, only there's just one item on the menu for each meal! That menu has been designed to balance your insulin and glucagon levels, bring down blood sugar levels, and make you feel wonderful! The meals include interesting foods you may not have enjoyed in the past (the average American eats the same twenty foods every day of his or her life). Now you've been given the opportunity to experiment with your taste buds and lose weight in the process.

This is the menu design I present to each of my weight-loss counseling clients, and I ask them to follow the program as precisely as they can. It will take some adjustment on your part, but that's what you expected, isn't it? After all, if you keep eating the way you have been eating, you'll weigh what you've always weighed!

> *"It was this program that made it possible for me to make it through the holidays and stay on track the whole time."*
> **MARY**

You may find the occasional meal you really don't enjoy. At those times you may substitute the menu for one from another day. Many of the meals that follow can be completely prepared several days in advance and simply reheated a few minutes before you need to set dinner on the table. Make Saturday your cooking day, for example. To cut down on meal preparation time, we recommend that you use leftovers for your lunch meal. Every recipe can be stored in the refrigerator for a short period of time; most can be frozen to be enjoyed at a later date.

While you may have a favorite recipe similar to the recipes found here, please don't substitute! We've planned these menus and recipes carefully to conform to the balance that is the whole premise of this book, so be open-minded!

What follows is a thirty-day menu plan. I've included the meal replacement bar or drink for the morning meal, because you'll find it easier to comply with the program if you don't have to think about breakfast. If you simply *must* eat a "normal" breakfast occasionally, try your favorite egg recipe with just a little carbohydrate (one-half rice cake or one-half apple) on the side. It will work just fine.

By the way, please read our section on supplementation in chapter 9. You will need to include a fine-quality multivitamin/mineral complex each day to ensure that you're receiving all the micronutrients you need for optimum health. The supplementation is an important part of the program.

a month's worth of menus

Over the years I have found that most people like the structure of being told exactly what to eat. They don't want to have to figure it out—especially when they're trying to make such a dramatic shift in their eating lifestyle. So in this introductory period, please do not deviate from these menus. They have been balanced for macronutrient content.

After you work with the menus for a while, you'll soon figure out how to balance foods for yourself. Think of the following menus as a set of "training wheels" to get you started. The page number beside each new entrée refers to the recipe for that dish in Appendix A.

Day 1

Breakfast: Breakfast bar or protein drink (p. 198)
Lunch: Large serving of the Basic Salad (p. 238), topped with canned tuna fish (okay to use tuna canned in spring water).
Dinner: Lemon Pepper Halibut (p. 263), Steamed Rice (p. 281), Roasted Asparagus (p. 275), 1 small piece of Pumpkin Pie (p. 295)
Snack (optional): Roasted, Toasted Pumpkin Seeds (p. 291)

Day 2

Breakfast: Breakfast bar or protein drink

Lunch: Leftover Lemon Pepper Halibut with one serving of the Basic Salad

Dinner: Itsa Meatball (p. 266), Baby Greens Salad with Basil Vinaigrette (p. 240)

Snack (optional): Avocado Salad (p. 288)

Day 3

Breakfast: Breakfast bar or protein drink

Lunch: Leftover Itsa Meatball with large serving of the Baby Greens Salad

Dinner: Black Bean Chili (p. 245), *small piece* of Wheat-Free Corn Bread with a little butter (p. 287)

Snack (optional): Almond butter stuffed into a celery stalk

Day 4

Breakfast: Breakfast bar or protein drink

Lunch: Leftover Black Bean Chili

Dinner: Roasted Chicken with Mushroom Gravy (p. 273), Roasted Vegetables (p. 275), *small piece* of Wheat-Free Corn Bread (p. 287)

Snack (optional): Chicken Pâté (p. 289)

Day 5

Breakfast: Breakfast bar or protein drink

Lunch: Leftover Roasted Chicken with Mushroom Gravy, Roasted Vegetables

Dinner: Mock Filet Mignon (p. 267), Sautéed Zucchini (p. 278), *small piece* of Pumpkin Pie (p. 295)

Snack (optional): Sinful Deviled Eggs (p. 290)

Day 6

Breakfast: Breakfast bar or protein drink

Lunch: Leftover Mock Filet Mignon with large serving of the Basic Salad

Dinner: Cider-Poached Cod with Caramelized Onions (p. 258), Sautéed Broccoli (p. 277), and portion of the Basic Salad

Snack (optional): Buffalo Chicken Wings (p. 289)

Day 7

Breakfast: Breakfast bar or protein drink

Lunch: Portion of the Basic Salad topped with leftover Cider-Poached Cod with Caramelized Onions

Dinner: Apple Cider Chicken (p. 249), Roasted Vegetables (p. 275), and Pasta Side Dish (p. 272)

Snack (optional): 1 tablespoon roasted or raw sesame seeds

Day 8

Breakfast: Breakfast bar or protein drink

Lunch: Leftover Apple Cider Chicken, leftover Roasted Vegetables

Dinner: Cioppino (p. 259), Wheat-Free Corn Bread with a small pat of butter (p. 287), Baby Greens Salad with Thyme Vinaigrette (p. 241)

Snack (optional): (See above snack options)

Day 9

Breakfast: Breakfast bar or protein drink

Lunch: Leftover Cioppino, leftover Baby Greens Salad with Thyme Vinaigrette (p. 241)

Dinner: Chicken and Mushroom Casserole (p. 256), Baby Greens Salad with Thyme Vinaigrette (p. 241), one small orange

Snack (optional): (See above snack options)

Day 10

Breakfast: Breakfast bar or protein drink

Lunch: Leftover Chicken and Mushroom Casserole, leftover Baby Greens Salad with Thyme Vinaigrette
Dinner: Pasta Primavera and Chicken with Red Sauce (p. 270), Baby Greens Salad with Red Pepper Vinaigrette (p. 243)
Snack (optional): (See above snack options)

Day 11

Breakfast: Breakfast bar or protein drink
Lunch: Leftover Pasta Primavera and Chicken with Red Sauce, Baby Greens Salad with Red Pepper Vinaigrette
Dinner: Lentil Soup with Herbs (p. 283), 3–4 ounces Roasted Turkey Breast (p. 274) (or other leftover protein), pear or other small fruit
Snack (optional): (See above snack options)

Day 12

Breakfast: Breakfast bar or protein drink
Lunch: Leftover Lentil Soup with Herbs, with 3–4 ounces of Roasted Turkey Breast (or other leftover protein)
Dinner: Crab Cakes with Lemon Caper Sauce (p. 260), Baby Baby Greens Salad with Dill Vinaigrette (p. 242), small portion of Fresh Veggies (p. 276)
Snack (optional): (See above snack options)

Day 13

Breakfast: Breakfast bar or protein drink
Lunch: Leftover Crab Cakes with Lemon Caper Sauce, leftover Fresh Veggies
Dinner: Shepherd's Pie (p. 281)
Snack (optional): (See above snack options)

Day 14

Breakfast: Breakfast bar or protein drink

Lunch: Leftover Shepherd's Pie
Dinner: Seasoned Beef in Corn Tortillas (p. 265)
Snack (optional): (See above snack options)

Day 15

Breakfast: Breakfast bar or protein drink
Lunch: Leftover Seasoned Beef in Corn Tortillas
Dinner: Stuffed Filet of Sole (p. 264), leftover Baby Greens Salad
with Dill Vinaigrette (p. 242), Pasta Side Dish (p. 272)
Snack (optional): (See above snack options)

Day 16

Breakfast: Breakfast bar or protein drink
Lunch: Leftover Stuffed Filet of Sole, leftover Pasta Side Dish
Dinner: Roasted Chicken with Mushroom Gravy (p. 273), Baked
Potato Without Fat (p. 248), tiny portion of the Basic Salad or
Baby Greens Salad with Dill Vinaigrette
Snack (optional): (See above snack options)

Day 17

Breakfast: Breakfast bar or protein drink
Lunch: Leftover Roasted Chicken with Mushroom Gravy, large
portion of the Basic Salad
Dinner: Tortilla Chicken Soup (p. 285)
Snack (optional): (See above snack options)

Day 18

Breakfast: Breakfast bar or protein drink
Lunch: Leftover Tortilla Chicken Soup
Dinner: Roasted Turkey Breast (p. 274), Roasted Asparagus (p.
275), Baked Potato Without Fat, Orange Date Bars (p. 294)
Snack (optional): (See above snack options)

Day 19

Breakfast: Breakfast bar or protein drink
Lunch: Leftover Roasted Turkey Breast, leftover Roasted Asparagus
Dinner: Salisbury Steak (p. 268), Baked Potato Without Fat, large portion of the Basic Salad
Snack (optional): (See above snack options)

Day 20

Breakfast: Breakfast bar or protein drink
Lunch: Leftover Salisbury Steak, large portion of the Basic Salad
Dinner: Baked Snapper with Spicy Black Beans (p. 257), small portion of Baby Greens Salad
Snack (optional): (See above snack options)

Day 21

Breakfast: Breakfast bar or protein drink
Lunch: Leftover Baked Snapper with Spicy Black Beans, Baby Greens Salad
Dinner: Grandma's Turkey Soup (p. 282)
Snack (optional): (See above snack options)

Day 22

Breakfast: Breakfast bar or protein drink
Lunch: Leftover Grandma's Turkey Soup
Dinner: Chicken and Brown Rice Casserole (p. 250), Sautéed Broccoli (p. 277), 1 small orange
Snack (optional): (See above snack options)

Day 23

Breakfast: Breakfast bar or protein drink
Lunch: Leftover Chicken and Brown Rice Casserole, leftover Sautéed Broccoli, small serving of fruit

Dinner: Chinese Chicken Salad (p. 253)
Snack (optional): (See above snack options)

Day 24

Breakfast: Breakfast bar or protein drink
Lunch: Leftover Chinese Chicken Salad
Dinner: Southwestern Chili (p. 284), small apple
Snack (optional): (See above snack options)

Day 25

Breakfast: Breakfast bar or protein drink
Lunch: Leftover Southwestern Chili, with apple
Dinner: Chicken Tacos (p. 251)
Snack (optional): (See above snack options)

Day 26

Breakfast: Breakfast bar or protein drink
Lunch: Leftover Chicken Tacos
Dinner: White Bean Minestrone (p. 286), Roasted Chicken Breast (p. 272)
Snack (optional): (See above snack options)

Day 27

Breakfast: Breakfast bar or protein drink
Lunch: Leftover White Bean Minestrone, canned tuna fish moistened with 1 tablespoon mayonnaise
Dinner: Thai Vegetables with Chicken (p. 278), Steamed Rice (p. 281), small apple
Snack (optional): (See above snack options)

Day 28

Breakfast: Breakfast bar or protein drink
Lunch: Leftover Thai Vegetables with Chicken, small apple

Dinner: Curried Seafood Stew (p. 262), Steamed Rice (p. 281), Roasted Asparagus (p. 275)

Snack (optional): (See above snack options)

Day 29

Breakfast: Breakfast bar or protein drink

Lunch: Leftover Curried Seafood Stew, leftover Roasted Asparagus

Dinner: Chicken Enchilada Casserole (p. 254), Sautéed Green and Yellow Beans (p. 277), small portion of The Basic Salad

Snack (optional): (See above snack options)

Day 30

Breakfast: Breakfast bar or protein drink

Lunch: Leftover Chicken Enchilada Casserole, small portion of the Basic Salad

Dinner: Sesame Chicken with Stir-Fried Vegetables (p. 280), small serving of Pan-Fried Soba Noodles (p. 269)

Snack (optional): (See above snack options)

Day 31

Breakfast: Breakfast bar or protein drink

Lunch: Leftover Sesame Chicken with Stir-Fried Vegetables, small serving of leftover Pan-Fried Soba Noodles

Dinner: Black Bean Soup (p. 246)

Snack (optional): (See above snack options)

AT THE END OF THIRTY-ONE DAYS

How are you doing? You've been on the program for thirty-one days now, and you've had plenty of time to put the program to the test. Were you able to follow the menus? Did you enjoy the recipes? Were you able to clean your cupboard of all the non-foods and just eat according to the plan?

Are you losing weight? Is your energy high? Are you feeing more "balanced"? Are you noticing an increased feeling of well-being each day you are on the program? Does your body love what you are doing?

Most people on this program can answer yes to each of these questions. They're feeling "more balanced"; they do find that their energy level has improved—that they simply feel good in whatever sense that means for them; and yes, they're losing weight.

> *"I enjoyed how easy it was to follow this program and I can't say enough wonderful things about the menu."*
> **JANE**

For the next thirty days, I encourage you to recycle these menus. Don't do any experimentation on your own just yet; you simply haven't given the program enough time to become an in-grained part of your eating habits. In these menus you have thirty days of variety to enjoy. Make use of them!

Let's continue with the discussion of what to expect on this program. How much weight can you reasonably expect to lose? What if things aren't going quite the way you expected, and how can we turn this around for you? Let's talk about it.

What to Expect on This Food Plan

9

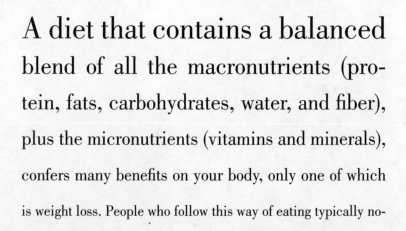

A diet that contains a balanced blend of all the macronutrients (protein, fats, carbohydrates, water, and fiber), plus the micronutrients (vitamins and minerals), confers many benefits on your body, only one of which is weight loss. People who follow this way of eating typically notice an immediate increase in energy, and they sleep better at night. Headaches often disappear, and other aches and pains diminish as highly allergenic foods disappear from the diet. This process may take a few weeks, but a reduced tendency toward what I call "fleeting inflammations" (inflammations in various parts of the body) is a common "side effect" of this balanced eating program.

Over the next few weeks, hair and fingernails grow faster and healthier; peeling and cracking of the fingernails disappear, and the nails themselves are stronger. Because of the addition of healthy fats, both men and women often notice that their skin is softer and moister, and they aren't wrinkling as fast. Many women find that their hormones are becoming more balanced as they provide their bodies with the nutrients they need to synthesize the sex hormones. Nearly everyone reports a renewed sense of well-being, of improved stamina, of new mental clarity.

Weight loss can be sudden at first; five to fifteen pounds often drop off within the first four weeks as excess water weight held in the tissues by insulin is discarded and a little fat weight is lost. After the initial drop, weight loss typically settles down to about one to two pounds per week. Even though this may seem slow, especially for those who have a significant amount of weight to lose, fat tissue cannot be burned more quickly than that! One to two pounds of fat loss each week is the *ideal* rate of weight loss. If you lose weight more quickly, you may be losing muscle tissue. If that is the case, I encourage you to increase the amount of protein you are enjoying each day by just five grams per day, and increase your workout program so that you can build strong, healthy muscle.

No matter how wonderful, how well-balanced, *how nourishing* this program is, some people's initial reactions are not always pleasant. Because so many of my clients have indulged freely in sugar and carbonated beverages for years and are literally addicted to them, they may experience at least three days of "withdrawal" with varying degrees of discomfort. Sally sat for three days on the floor of her living room without the energy to get up. Mark shook for two days, so full of anxiety and "nerves" that he had difficulty working or concentrating. Judy complained of headaches, as did several others. They had to force themselves to go on with the program for a few days until their withdrawal symptoms disappeared. It often takes three days to get past the unpleasantness and withdrawal and start feeling good. Be patient and stick to it. These three days will pass quickly.

> *"I get compliments regularly now from those who know me on how great I look."*
> **JORDAN**

The important thing to remember is this: You didn't gain your weight overnight, and you won't lose it overnight. Be patient with yourself. As you continue to follow this program, your health will continue to improve, day after day, week after week, year after year. You'll be able to look back and see continuous, steady progress in the accomplishment of your health goals. You will lose weight, and if you continue to follow the program, you will keep it off forever.

After a few weeks on the program, you may have questions about how you're feeling. Here are some of the most frequently asked questions and the concerns my clients express.

Question 1: *I'm following your diet plan carefully, but I still find myself getting hungry in the late afternoon. Why?*

Answer: There are usually three reasons people become hungry on this program.

A. You may not be eating enough food. You may have calculated your protein requirements incorrectly and simply need more food just to satisfy your daily calorie requirement. In that case, increase your protein, your carbohydrates, and your fat proportionately! Do not be tempted to throw in a high-carb snack between meals (like an apple or bag of popcorn, for example). You may find it particularly helpful to add a *well-balanced snack* midafternoon or before you go to bed. Check the recipe section in Appendix A for excellent snack suggestions. Your meals should be spaced about four to five hours apart, no longer. If you have to wait longer than that to eat because of your schedule, plan a snack to fill in the gap. There is absolutely no reason to feel hungry on this program. Hunger will not increase or speed up weight loss.

B. The most common reason for hunger is that you are still consuming too many carbohydrates. Keep a food diary for a few days and analyze your meal history. Restrict your carbohydrates a little more and see if the hunger doesn't abate. Give your body about two or three days to balance itself.

C. Your body may need time to adjust. Sometimes your food allergies kick up a fuss by making you hungry when you eliminate them from your dinner plate. It's a false hunger. Learn to listen to your body. Give yourself a few days to get past the allergy; the hunger and other unpleasant symptoms will disappear soon.

Question 2: *I still experience an energy drain in the late afternoon about 4:00 p.m. Why?*

Answer: Either you are eating a meal that is too high in carbohydrates for lunch or breakfast, or you are eating a food to which you are allergic. Pay careful attention to wheat and dairy products. They typically cause inappropriate sleepiness or fatigue. Keep a food diary for a few days and see if you can discover which food is causing this energy drop. Make sure your meals contain enough protein and that your meals are not too high in carbohydrates.

If you have to wait too long between meals (longer than four hours or so), you may need to grab a little snack between meals to keep up your blood sugar. Some excellent snack foods are raw almonds or other raw nuts and seeds—a good choice is pumpkin seeds. A small handful of raw or roasted pumpkin seeds will often take away the need to munch on something crunchy and restore your energy level. Don't worry about the fat content; it's the beneficial kind of fat we've already talked about.

Question 3: *I'm constipated on this diet. Help!*

Answer: Let's look at several possibilities:

A. You may be consuming a food to which you are reacting; i.e., a wheat or dairy product. If you are still eating some grains or dairy products, try to eliminate them totally from your diet for a few days and see if the problem resolves itself. Both are common causes of constipation.

B. You may not be drinking enough water. Try increasing your water consumption to eight to ten glasses each day. Make sure you are drinking the water between meals.

C. You may not be eating enough fiber. Make sure you are eating at least five to six servings of raw or lightly steamed vegetables per day, in balance with your protein. The menu suggestions include several servings of vegetables each day. If you find that you simply can't do this, use a sugar-free fiber supplement with an additional eight ounces of water. Take the fiber supplement before you go to bed each night at least three hours after your last meal.

D. Certain mineral deficiencies can cause constipation, particularly deficiencies in magnesium and potassium. Use a magnesium supplement (not magnesium oxide) to increase your magnesium intake to about 500 milligrams per day. Take about 99 milligrams of potassium per day. (Avoid potassium chloride. Use both a magnesium and potassium ion bonded to an amino acid combination, or use magnesium glycinate. These mineral forms are typically well absorbed.) And remember that magnesium helps reduce craving for chocolate and sweets.

E. After following these suggestions, if you still can't get things moving again, you may need to resort temporarily to an herbal laxative that contains dandelion root, burdock, ginger, fennel, buckthorn, and small amounts of cascara sagrada. Sometimes it helps to take an herbal fiber supplement with psyllium husks and other fibers. *Be sure to drink plenty of water with them!*

Avoid all herbal laxatives that contain senna or large amounts of cascara sagrada. Most reputable herbal com-

recommended dietary supplement program

MULTIVITAMIN/MINERAL SUPPLEMENT

Choose a well-balanced supplement that contains significant amounts of both vitamins and minerals, including the trace minerals. I call this the "supplement foundation." Your supplement should contain virtually all nutrients known to be essential for human health. This will of necessity *NOT* be a one-a-day, because manufacturers simply cannot squeeze biologically significant amounts of all nutrients into one little tablet. You will be taking from two to four capsules per day *minimum*, just with your foundation piece—the multivitamin/mineral.

Make sure this foundation piece contains a well-rounded blend of both beta-carotene and vitamin A (around 15,000 to 25,000 IUs of beta carotene per dose), balanced B complex, from 500 to 1,000 milligrams of vitamin C, 100 IUs of vitamin D to enhance calcium absorption, 200 IUs of vitamin E, and a significant amount of all the minerals. The minerals should include calcium, magnesium, potassium, zinc, copper, iron, vanadium, chromium, selenium, boron, and about twenty of the trace minerals.

I usually recommend that you select the capsule form instead of the tablet form; many tablets can be difficult to swallow and unless your digestion is optimum, a tablet may not break down adequately in your stomach. Because of the encapsulation process, you will need to take a few more capsules than tablets to get the dosage you require, but in the long run, you'll benefit from the extra trouble.

There are several excellent multivitamin supplements

on the market available through your local health food store, GNC, or by calling the toll-free numbers in Appendix C. Some excellent brands are Nature's Life, Source Naturals, Eclectic Institute, TwinLab, PREVAIL, Nature's Secret, Country Life, Enzymatic Therapy, Solaray, and the Nutritionist Series.

OTHER MINERALS

Calcium: Up to 1,000 milligrams per day. Do not use calcium carbonate, oyster shell, bonemeal, dolomite, eggshell, or other inorganic sources of calcium. Use calcium citrate, amino acid chelates, or calcium bonded to other amino acids. Many of the above companies provide excellent selections. Check Appendix C for more information on how to obtain these products.

Magnesium: Up to 1,000 milligrams per day. Do not use magnesium oxide. Use magnesium glycinate, magnesium citrate, an amino acid chelate, or magnesium bonded to other amino acids. Many of the above companies provide excellent selections.

Zinc: Up to fifty milligrams per day. Use either zinc picolinate or a zinc bonded to amino acids. Many of the above companies provide an excellent selection.

Chromium: Up to 800 micrograms per day. Use either chromium picolinate or GTF chromium. Many of the above companies provide an excellent selection.

Iron: Only use additional iron if you do not include red meat in your diet or if you have followed a vegetarian diet for

(continued on page 220)

(continued from page 219)

a period of time, if you experience heavy bleeding during your menstrual cycle or have lost blood for other reasons, or if you have been diagnosed as iron deficient by your physician. Use no more than fifteen milligrams per day and do not use iron (or ferrous) fumerate, ferrous sulfate, or other inorganic sources of iron. Use iron citrate or an iron bonded to amino acids, along with additional vitamin C for maximum absorption. Many of the above companies provide an excellent selection.

Essential Fatty Acids: To make up for years of an EFA-deficient diet, it is recommended that you use from two to four tablespoons of raw oil, preferably flaxseed oil, each day. This oil must be purchased fresh and kept refrigerated at all times to avoid rancidity. You may also purchase flaxseed oil capsules if you prefer. If you are using at least two tablespoons of olive oil per day (in your salad dressing, for example), you will only need two tablespoons of flaxseed oil per day (about six capsules). Excellent sources include Barlean's, Nature's Life, and Country Life.

Some people also find great benefit from using evening primrose oil as part of their EFA program. From three to six capsules will suffice for most people. Remember, you have to eat fat to lose fat!

panies have formulated an herbal laxative that will stimulate the bowels without creating dependence on them.

Question 4: *If I eat perfectly on this plan, will I need to take dietary supplements?*

Answer: Although this plan is beautifully balanced among the macronutrients, there is no way you can receive the amount of micronutrients you need on a diet that is less than several *thousand* calories a day. Obviously this menu plan does not fit that category. More and more studies are proving what many of us have known for years: We need supplemental nutrition, given our stress levels, our poor dietary history (past deficiencies), the diminished quality of the food items we purchase in the supermarkets, environmental pollutants, and the other side effects of civilization.

This is particularly true for those individuals who have dieted frequently over the years. Reducing diets are so lacking in the micronutrients that are essential for human health that significant health challenges accompany those long-standing deficiencies. They simply will not be resolved by wishful thinking or adding a synthetic one-a-day vitamin.

I put all my clients on a comprehensive supplement program to meet their current needs and to correct past deficiencies. When I meet face-to-face with a client, I can write a program that is specific to his or her needs, but in this forum I will need to make some generalizations. Please keep in mind that this program may need to be fine-tuned to meet your personal needs.

You're probably saying, "I'm going to be spending a lot of money on supplements!" Yes, you will. I wish there were an easier, cheaper way to bring your body into nutritional balance, but there isn't. The truth is grim: Most Americans are seriously undernourished, and no group is at greater risk than dieters. You have been slowly starving your body to death over the years; you cannot recuperate overnight, even with the most perfect diet and the most perfect lifestyle.

You do not need to spend hundreds of dollars per month in supplements, however. Some inferior products are extremely expensive; others are extremely inexpensive. However, follow this one rule: High-quality supplements can seldom be found in a grocery, drugstore, discount store, or mail-order house. They are seldom found in the multilevel market industry. You will be told from time to time: "Just buy the cheapest vitamin on the market; they're all the same." That simply isn't true. While you don't need to pay megabucks, you can't pay microbucks either. You need to educate yourself on the subject of supplemental nutrition. Use the recommendations in this section to evaluate your products. Develop a relationship with the staff at your local health food store, and read, read, read! Purchase some reference books on nutrition and study the subject. Learn how to nourish your body!

Question 5: *My body doesn't feel good eating all that protein. I felt better when I was eating more fruits and grains.*

Answer: This is not a high-protein diet, so you are not eating more protein than your body requires if you follow our recommendations for protein requirements. The problem, therefore, is not that you're getting too much protein; it's that you're not able to digest it and use it. There may be a couple of reasons for this.

You may be deficient in zinc. The enzymes that digest protein contain zinc. If you have been zinc deficient for a period of time (if you have used a low-animal-protein diet for some time), you may lose your ability to digest protein. Protein foods just won't "feel" right to you. In my clinical experience, I have often correlated zinc deficiency with a distaste for protein and with cravings for carbohydrates. When the zinc deficiency was corrected, the clients acquired a "taste" for protein foods. Try including more zinc in your supplement program (up to 50 milligrams per day). You will not correct your zinc deficiency overnight, however; ex-

recommended reading guide

Prescription for Nutritional Healing, by Dr. James Balch, M.D., and Mrs. Phyllis Balch, C.C.N. Available in most health food stores. One of the best all-around guides to natural health. Easy to use.

The Real Vitamin and Mineral Book, by Shari Liebermann, Ph.D. Highly recommended. Lists every nutrient individually and gives optimum dosage levels for each one.

The Big Family Guide to All the Vitamins, by Ruth Adams. Excellent reference source for information on vitamins and how to use them.

The Nutrition Desk Reference, by Robert Garrison, Jr., and Elizabeth Somer.

The Big Family Guide to All the Minerals, by Frank Murray. An excellent source for information on minerals and how to use them.

These books are available in most health food stores, or GNC, or can be special-ordered for you. See Appendix C for information on how to obtain them locally.

pect to get better and better results over a period of eight to twelve weeks.

Meanwhile, gradually increase the amount of protein you are using, as you are comfortable, until you have reached the amount of protein that is optimum for you. At the same time, reduce the starches from your diet so that you're starting to bring your

> *"The secret to permanent
> weight loss is dietary
> balance; balancing the
> protein, carbohydrate, and
> fat at every meal. You need
> never gain weight again!"*
> **CAROL SIMONTACCHI**

protein-to-carbohydrate ratios into balance to reduce the secretion of insulin.

As your body adjusts to higher and higher levels of protein, it will begin to secrete more of the enzymes it needs to digest the protein, another part of your body's natural homeostatic tendency. Within a short period of time, you will again find that you can digest and use the protein.

You may benefit from using supplemental plant enzymes that contain protease (to digest protein), lipase (to digest fats), or pancreatic enzymes. Some excellent companies that manufacture digestive enzymes include Enzymatic Therapy, Nature's Life, PREVAIL, and Source Naturals. These supplements can be purchased from your local health food store, GNC, or consult Appendix C for instructions on how to obtain them. Follow the instructions on the bottle.

Remember to chew your foods carefully. Relax before your meals. Don't eat when you are upset or nervous. Sip a cup of ginger tea (or chew on some raw ginger) just before dinner to stimulate digestive juices. Use digestive bitters (available from your local health food store) to stimulate the liver and pancreas. Don't drink too much liquid during the meal (you should drink your eight to ten glasses of water mostly between meals so your digestive juices are not diluted).

Question 6: *I'm afraid my cholesterol will go through the roof on this diet. Isn't a more vegetarian diet healthier for my heart and arteries?*

Answer: This is one of the first questions I'm usually asked when I teach this concept. And the answer is simple: No! This diet is so well-balanced that your cholesterol and triglycerides will also become more balanced.

A healthy liver produces the amount of cholesterol equivalent to over eighty pats of butter—every day. Dietary cholesterol is relatively insignificant in terms of serum cholesterol, but even elevated serum cholesterol does not become a problem until it oxidizes Fats become rancid in the body when exposed to oxygen, just as fats become rancid sitting in your kitchen cabinet. This rancidity is called oxidation. Preventing the oxidation of blood fats is a simple matter of eating more fruits and vegetables that provide a rich supply of antioxidant nutrients and using supplemental vitamin C or other antioxidants.

If we look at the hormone issue again, we see that the very hormone responsible for producing excessive cholesterol (HMG CoA reductase) is triggered by excessive insulin—another important reason to keep insulin levels low. Elevated triglycerides are triggered primarily by the excessive consumption of sugars. Numerous studies have shown that triglycerides can be brought down simply by including more seafood in the diet (our menu plan provides several portions of fish each week) and by eating more fiber-rich vegetables than we're accustomed to eating.

We have to look at protein/carbohydrate/fat balance as more than just a weight-loss technique. Balancing the diet appropriately confers tremendous health benefits on every part of the body. It is a heart-healthy, brain-healthy diet. No wonder we feel so good on it!

> *"Just because we're fat*
> *doesn't mean we're mentally*
> *or emotionally or spiritually*
> *sick. It usually means that*
> *we simply haven't been*
> *taught how to eat*
> *to stay slim."*
> **CAROL SIMONTACCHI**

Question 7: *I just don't have time to prepare all these meals. It's easier for me if I can just whip up something in a hurry. How can I adapt this eating plan to my lifestyle?*

Answer: This is a tough question and easier to discuss than to do. What the questions infers is this: "I haven't made a place in my life for nourishing my body. My health takes second place to everything else I *want* to do."

We Americans have strayed further and further from the art of nurturing ourselves, to the point that our health is suffering. At some point, we're all going to have to reevaluate our goals and restructure our lives to *make* time for this all-important activity. We simply aren't going to be able to pull just anything off the grocery shelf and expect it to fulfill our health needs. We need to make some lifestyle changes.

At the same time, we all have to earn a living. Many of us have young children at home, and we want to devote every possible moment to their care. We don't want to spend our precious time "slaving over a hot stove" when we could relax some of our priorities and have more fun with the kids. Here are some simple suggestions for making this program work for you:

A. Make your breakfast the simplest meal of the day.

B. Plan your menus at least one week in advance. Don't leave anything to the last minute. After planning your menus, do your grocery shopping on a day when your schedule permits a more relaxed shopping experience (by the way, don't shop when you're hungry; you'll be tempted by those things you shouldn't eat), and do as much advance preparation as you can.

There is much you can do on a Saturday morning, for instance, to make your meal preparation during the following week much easier. Follow our salad-making instructions and prepare most of the vegetables when you bring them home from the grocery store. Dry them carefully and store them in food storage bags in the refrigerator.

Every meal that you can make ahead and freeze, *do it!* Go through your menus, choose which ones are easily frozen, and prepare them on the weekend. Freeze them in portion sizes so all you have to do is defrost and reheat. Make as many of these dishes as you can. Especially good for a quick meal are the chili and bean soup recipes.

Keep raw nuts and seeds on hand for quick munchies. Keep these in your car so you're not tempted to stop at a fast-food restaurant when you're hungry. Or use one of the meal replacement bars we recommended earlier. Carry a bottle of water with you at all times so you won't drink soft drinks when you're thirsty.

Are you picking up on a general theme here? *The key to success is preparation!*

C. If you are the food shopper in the family, buy only those foods that you can eat. Don't feel that you need to indulge your spouse and children by buying them junk foods. If the food isn't good for you, it isn't good for them. They will benefit from the same eating program you are developing for yourself.

If you don't buy it, it won't be in the house, and you won't be tempted in a moment of weakness. Are you picking up on another theme here? *Take charge of your pantry!*

D. Get someone to watch over you. My clients repeatedly tell me how important it is for them to be accountable to someone. Who can you be accountable to? Can you organize a weight-loss group among your neighbors or friends? Will your spouse take the responsibility of making sure you are complying with the program and offer encouragement when you're feeling discouraged? Can you get a group together in the office? Can you find a small group of friends with whom you can exercise and discuss your program? Remember: What you are accountable for gets done!

Those of you who are moms and dads know about the importance of holding your children accountable for their schoolwork or chores. If you simply say, "Jerry, go clean your room," and you go on to something else, chances are good Jerry will simply ignore the instruction. But if you say, "I'll be checking on your job in thirty minutes . . . ," and you follow through a few times, Jerry will be more responsive to your instructions.

We may be thirty or forty years older than our Jerry, but we aren't so much more mature! We tend to accomplish what we're accountable for. Find someone who will hold you to your resolve and help you succeed.

Question 8: *I'm getting unbelievable cravings for sweets or chocolate. I can't stay away from bread. What am I doing wrong?*

Answer: You're not doing anything wrong. It isn't your lack of self-control that's driving the passion for a certain food. There can be a number of reasons your food cravings and bingeing occasionally get out of control. Again, the answer lies deep in your endocrine system and in a disordered mineral balance. Your body is talking to you, trying to get your attention. It's saying, "I need some minerals!" Although food allergies can contribute to cravings for certain foods (see chapter 3), several minerals play a key role in reducing or eliminating food cravings. When they are added into the diet appropriately, it seems almost like magic how the cravings go away.

Just can't stop thinking about that box of chocolate chip cookies your kids hid in the freezer? Planning to take a quick trip into town for a quart of pistachio ice cream? Could you just die for a piece of French bread, preferably smothered in garlic butter, or a plate of pasta topped with white clam sauce? Here are some suggestions for what mineral supplements to add to your diet when the munchies hit.

Craving for bread or pasta? Zinc Picolinate (up to 50 milligrams a day)

Craving for salty foods? Drink ginseng tea—Siberian, Korean, or American—or use standardized extract of ginseng root. Use vitamin C (1,000 milligrams a day) with pantothenic acid (100–500 milligrams a day). You may also use licorice root tea with the ginseng.

Craving for crunchy foods? Slice jicama or carrots very thin and enjoy ice cold with your favorite dressing. Or try Roasted, Toasted Pumpkin Seeds (p. 291)

(continued on page 230)

(continued from page 229)

Craving for fatty foods? Eat a tablespoon of raw almond or other nut butters right off the spoon (yes, it's decadent!). Slice ripe avocado thin, dress with an olive oil/lemon juice dressing, and enjoy!

Craving for carbonated beverages? Use unsweetened sparkling mineral water, flavored with freshly squeezed lemon or lime juice.

Craving for alcohol? L-Glutamine (1,000–2,000 milligrams a day on an empty stomach, along with the herbs gymnema sylvestre and kudzu (available through your local health food store or check Appendix C for information on obtaining the products).

Craving for chocolate? Magnesium Glycinate, Citrate, or Aspartate (up to 1,000 milligrams a day or until you experience diarrhea).

Craving for sweets of any type? Add magnesium (up to 1,000 milligrams a day), zinc (up to 50 milligrams a day), and chromium (up to 800 micrograms a day).

If you are still unable to control your cravings for sugars, consider using the Enique International Eat Away lozenge. I developed this lozenge for certain individuals in response to their struggle to break their addiction to sugar. It contains a blend of amino acids and herbs that not only remove sugar craving but make it virtually *impossible* to enjoy sugary treats! The lozenge also takes away the appetite for one to two hours (excellent for that midafternoon grazing period). Check Appendix C for more information on how to obtain this product.

Question 9: *I eat when I'm depressed, angry, or discouraged. How can I break this habit?*

Answer: The first step in breaking this habit is recognizing that you do it. You eat for reasons other than nourishing your body. Once you've acknowledged this, you're well on your way toward developing healthy eating habits.

Second, you need to find out what is *really* bothering you. Why are you depressed or angry? Why are you discouraged? Can you talk about your feelings with someone? We often experience deep emotions because our emotional centers are trying to put certain situations into perspective and lay them to rest. Learn to be introspective so that you can help your mind do its own job of inner healing. You may need to consult a professional if you can't seem to pinpoint what's bothering you.

The second step is to make healthy substitutions. When you're desperate to eat something inappropriate, it does no good to grit your teeth and bolster your resolve. You simply aren't that tough. Eat something, but first ask yourself what you would really enjoy. You don't have to eat a cookie to satisfy all your cravings, you know. Try a cup of herbal tea with a handful of raw almonds or pumpkin seeds. Or maybe you would enjoy some barbecued chicken wings or a cup of cottage cheese piled into a quarter of a juicy ripe melon. If you truly practice eating the balanced plan I'm advocating, including the use of vitamin and mineral supplementation, you will begin to lose your taste for the old way of eating, and you won't ever want to return to it.

> *"I'm healed on the inside for
> the first time since I was
> a child."*
> ETTA

Maybe a nonfood activity will satisfy that inner itch. You may enjoy brisk walking in the park or woods, reading a book out on the patio, playing a game of golf . . . or badminton with your kids. Choose something you really enjoy doing and indulge yourself in an activity other than eating unhealthy foods.

The third and final step is to reward yourself for the great job you're doing. Remember, your eating and coping habits are as old as you are and may even reach back several generations. Don't expect to change forty years of habit overnight. When you've handled a situation correctly, do something really nice for yourself. Ask your spouse to give you a foot massage (or pay a professional for it!); soak in a hot tub bubbling with fragrant oil; enroll in an art class; spend a day fly-fishing; learn how to dance the rhumba; join a health club—whatever you can afford and enjoy, and *do it!* Life is not an endurance contest.

Question 10: *I keep trying to do everything right, but I cheat. I'm going to quit.*

Answer: Don't ever give up! If you really do blow it and go on an eating binge that doesn't end for a while, it's not the end of your program. Don't pull back into yourself and say, "See? I can't do it!" and shut the whole thing down. Instead, say to yourself, "Well, I blew it today. Tomorrow is another day and I'm back on the program." Pick up where you left off!

Let's face it: No matter how motivated you are, and no matter how clearly you understand the principles in this book, you are going to cheat from time to time. The deciding factor is what you do afterward. Judy just picked up where she left off. She didn't even gain a pound from her eating binge. Within twenty-four hours she was back on the program, and her weight continued to drop.

Another thing to remember is that whether or not you regain your weight or remain slim and trim is dependent upon cheating properly. If you cheat, at least do it well!

For example, you've been invited to a friend's house for dinner. You know she always serves chocolate cake and ice cream for dessert, and you don't want to offend her (not that you *want* to eat it, understand). You say, "It won't hurt just once . . ." The moment you say that, you stand at a crossroads: Eat the chocolate cake and keep eating the chocolate cake or eat the chocolate cake *balanced with additional protein* and get yourself immediately back on track. The easiest way to illustrate this point is through my own personal experience with cheating:

After being on this plan for about two weeks and having lost about four pounds, my husband and I went out for dinner. He said, "You've been really good on this diet. You can have a piece of cake for a treat tonight."

I thought about that and eyed the carrot cake lustfully. I thought, *He's right! I have been good.* The carrot cake was delicious.

Within one hour I started to get a headache. Three hours later I had a splitting headache and felt nauseated. By the time I got home, I was so sick I could hardly hold up my head. The next morning I was still so weak I could hardly stumble out of bed.

Here's what happened to me. Up to that point, my blood sugar was very steady, and the pancreas had decreased its release of insulin because it wasn't needing it. When my stomach took one "look" at the carrot cake approaching, it panicked and sent all kinds of messages to the pancreas: "We need insulin . . . hurry!" The pancreas responded instantly, totally out of proportion. The result was that insulin flooded my bloodstream, pulling glucose out of my bloodstream far in excess of what should have been pulled, and left my blood sugar drastically low. It took three days to get my glucose levels under control again. Believe me, that piece of carrot cake wasn't worth it.

Two weeks later my husband and I went out for dinner again, and he said, "You can have dessert tonight. It won't hurt you." (What a short memory!) This time I thought very carefully and finally said, "All right, I can have a piece of cake tonight, but only on one condition. That you not say anything about how I'm going to eat it."

He said he didn't care, so I ordered the cake with a cup of cottage cheese on the side. I ate them together—with no ill effects afterward!

Now please don't think you can spend the rest of your life in the cheat mode; but for those occasions when you really do want to have some extra carbohydrate (cake, cookie, pie) just calculate what protein you need to eat with it and indulge yourself. You really do deserve it once in a while.

My rule of thumb is dessert once a week. No more, no less! I just cheat properly.

> *"Let's face it: Our culture discriminates against fat people in their work, in their social lives, in their medical treatments, in every part of their lives."*
> **CAROL SIMONTACCHI**

IF YOU DON'T CHEAT PROPERLY

If you eat a lot of carbohydrates without the accompanying protein, your insulin levels will swing violently. Symptoms of insulin overload can be headache, nausea, light-headedness, extreme exhaustion. It isn't worth it.

If you do err on the side of too many carbohydrates and don't feel well, realize it will take a little time to regulate your blood sugar. Resume eating the way you've been instructed to by balancing the protein/carbohydrate/fat/water ratio, and let your body normalize itself again. You can't speed up the process by eating more protein and fewer carbohydrates. Just let your body do the work of restoring its balance.

ready, set, go!

We have addressed so many issues in the pages of this book that it's tempting to throw up your hands and say, "I can't even begin to do this! I don't know where to start!" We've talked about female issues and male issues; brown fat, insulin, and glucagon. We've talked about food allergies, nonfoods, and the thyroid. In short, we've brought the whole body into the conversation about what should be a simple discussion—weight loss. Many of these issues you will have to tackle one by one. Some of them your health care practitioner will need to address with you.

If there's just one message that you take away from all this material, it is this: Most of you did not choose to be overweight by gluttony or even poor food choices. Most of you eat the same food as just about everyone else. In a very real sense, *your fat is not your fault*. But this doesn't mean you have no options left. It doesn't mean you have to remain overweight.

The issues are quite complex, but I've given you the tools to get your life back in balance—to get your *diet* back in balance. Once you've restored balance, you can lose the weight *forever*.

And now, just think of today as Day 1. Today is the day you're going to start on your program. You're going to begin tackling the issues one by one. And pound by pound the excess weight will drop off for good.

> *"Obesity is seldom a case of overindulgence. It is almost never a case of sloth or gormandizing. Your fat really isn't your fault!"*
> CAROL SIMONTACCHI

Bon Appetit! Recipes for the No Fault/ No Fat Losers!

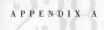
The Basic Salad

Serves 4

This "basic salad" should be part of your repertoire of salad recipes. While you may want to vary the selection of vegetables you enjoy in a salad, plan to use at least ten different varieties each time to provide the full spectrum of phytochemicals so beneficial to health. Use vegetables with bright hues of orange, red, purple, green, and yellow, and use as many seasonal vegetables as possible.

Don't be afraid to try these vegetables in the raw state! Raw foods are full of enzymes that help digest your food and provide your body with a wide variety of minerals and vitamins that improve your energy and the health of your whole body! You'll want to enjoy this salad several times per week.

1	clove garlic	¾	cup jicama*
1½	cups broccoli	1	cucumber
¾	cup onions, raw	¾	cup beets, raw
1½	bunches salad greens	¾	cup cauliflower
¾	cup zucchini, raw	2	tablespoons extra-virgin olive oil
1	stalk celery, raw		Juice of one lemon
1½	green onions		
1½	cups raw carrots		

It's a good idea to prepare all salad ingredients when you bring them home from the grocery store. Wash the greens carefully, dry them, and seal them in storage bags in the refrigerator. The other

---

*See Appendix B for more information about this product.

vegetables can be washed, peeled, and sealed in bags and stored in the refrigerator as well. They will keep well for several days.

At mealtime, mash the garlic clove with a fork and rub the inside of the salad bowl with it. Either leave it in the bowl or discard it. Prepare all salad ingredients and place them in the salad bowl. Toss gently. If you are going to enjoy the entire salad immediately, add the dressing to the whole salad. If you are going to save part of it for another meal, remove the portion to be saved and store in the refrigerator in a tightly covered container without dressing.

Lightly sprinkle the salad with the extra-virgin olive oil, and again toss gently but thoroughly to coat all the pieces with the oil. Rub the lemon firmly around on the table to break up the tissues inside, then cut it in half. Squeeze the juice over the salad with as much juice as you like. Toss again briefly to distribute the lemon juice, and serve immediately. For extra flavor, you may sprinkle an herbal seasoning on top of the salad.

Baby Greens Salad

Serves 4

1	clove garlic, chopped fine	2	cups cucumbers, peeled
1	tablespoon balsamic vinegar*	1⅓	cups radishes, sliced thin
2	tablespoons olive oil	1½	pounds mixed lettuce or mesclun mix*
⅔	cups Roma tomatoes		

*See Appendix B for more information about this product.

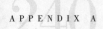

Vinaigrette

Whip together garlic and vinegar in a small bowl. Add olive oil slowly while continuing to whip. Season with salt and pepper to taste.

Quarter and slice Roma tomatoes and cucumbers. Mix together with the radishes and half of the vinaigrette. Let stand ten minutes. Mix together the lettuce and the rest of the dressing. Place on a plate and top with tomato, cucumber, and radish mixture. Serve immediately.

Meal-in-a-Flash Prep Plan

All vegetables can be cut up ahead of time, wrapped tightly, and refrigerated. Salad dressing can be made up to two weeks in advance, covered, and refrigerated.

Baby Greens Salad with Basil Vinaigrette

Serves 4

Who says salad should be boring? You'll want to make this simple salad a regular feature on your family's menu. Basil is an aromatic herb from Indonesia and India and is highly regarded as an herb that calms an upset stomach.

2	teaspoons fresh basil, chopped fine	⅔	cup Roma tomatoes
1	clove garlic, chopped fine	2	cups cucumbers, peeled
1	tablespoon balsamic vinegar	⅔	cup radishes, sliced thin
2	tablespoons olive oil	1½	pounds mixed lettuce or mesclun mix*

*See Appendix B for more information about this product.

Vinaigrette

Whip together the basil, garlic, and vinegar in a small bowl. Add olive oil slowly while continuing to whip. Season with salt and pepper.

Quarter and slice Roma tomatoes and cucumbers. Mix together with the radishes and half of the vinaigrette. Let stand ten minutes. Mix together the lettuce and rest of the dressing. Place on a plate and top with tomato, cucumber, and radish mixture. Serve immediately.

Meal-in-a-Flash Prep Plan

All vegetables can be cut up ahead of time, wrapped tightly, and refrigerated. Salad dressing can be made up to two weeks in advance, covered, and refrigerated.

Baby Greens Salad with Thyme Vinaigrette

Serves 4

Another delightful salad, with just a little different herb base! European herbalists used thyme to improve digestion and relieve chronic dyspepsia (indigestion).

2	tablespoons fresh thyme,* chopped finely	2	tablespoons olive oil
2	teaspoons garlic, chopped fine	⅔	cup Roma tomatoes
1	tablespoon balsamic vinegar*	2	cups cucumbers, peeled
		⅔	cup radishes, sliced thin
		1½	pounds mixed lettuce or mesclun mix*

*See Appendix B for more information about this product.

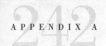

Vinaigrette

Whip together the thyme, garlic, and vinegar in a small bowl. Add olive oil slowly while continuing to whip. Season with salt and pepper.

Quarter and slice Roma tomatoes and cucumbers. Mix together with the radishes and half the vinaigrette. Let stand ten minutes. Mix together the lettuce and rest of dressing. Place on a plate and top with tomato, cucumber, and radish mixture. Serve immediately.

Meal-in-a-Flash Prep Plan

All vegetables can be cut up ahead of time, wrapped tightly, and refrigerated. Salad dressing can be made up to two weeks in advance, covered, and refrigerated.

Baby Greens Salad with Dill Vinaigrette

Serves 4

Fresh dill is available in most grocery stores year-round. Don't be tempted to use the dried seeds; they won't work in this recipe. You'll want to enjoy this aromatic fresh herb out of the garden.

2	*tablespoons fresh dill, chopped fine*	⅔	*cup Roma tomatoes*
2	*teaspoons garlic, chopped fine*	2	*cups cucumbers, peeled*
		⅔	*cup radishes, sliced thin*
1	*tablespoon lemon juice*	1½	*pounds mixed lettuce or mesclun mix**
2	*tablespoons olive oil*		

---

*See Appendix B for more information about this product.

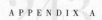

Vinaigrette

Whip together the dill, garlic, and lemon juice in a small bowl. Add olive oil slowly while continuing to whip. Season with salt and pepper.

Quarter and slice Roma tomatoes and cucumbers. Mix together with the radishes and half the vinaigrette. Let stand ten minutes. Mix together the lettuce and rest of dressing. Place on a plate and top with tomato, cucumber, and radish mixture. Serve immediately.

Meal-in-a-Flash Prep Plan

All vegetables can be cut up ahead of time, wrapped tightly, and refrigerated. Salad dressing can be a made up to two weeks in advance, covered, and refrigerated.

Baby Greens Salad with Red Pepper Vinaigrette

Serves 4

This is a very satisfying version of the Baby Greens Salad. The "fire" of the garlic is muted by the savory red pepper puree. And by the way, garlic is an excellent tonic for the cardiovascular and immune systems.

2	tablespoons roasted red bell peppers (canned, drained)	2	tablespoons olive oil
		⅔	cup Roma tomatoes
2	teaspoons garlic, chopped fine	2	cups cucumbers, peeled
		⅔	cup radishes, sliced thin
1	tablespoon balsamic vinegar*	1½	pounds mixed lettuce or mesclun mix*

*See Appendix B for more information about this product.

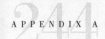

Vinaigrette

In a food process or blender, whip together the bell pepper, garlic, and vinegar. Add olive oil slowly while continuing to whip. Season with salt and pepper.

Quarter and slice Roma tomatoes and cucumbers. Mix together with the radishes and half the vinaigrette. Let stand ten minutes. Mix together the lettuce and rest of dressing. Place on a plate and top with tomato, cucumber, and radish mixture. Serve immediately.

Meal-in-a-Flash Prep Plan

All vegetables can be cut up ahead of time, wrapped tightly, and refrigerated. Salad dressing can be made up to two weeks in advance, covered, and refrigerated.

Garden Salad with Guacamole Dressing

Serves 4

You'll feel like you're cheating with this rich salad, but you're not! Avocado is a high-fat vegetable with the healthy fats that keep the skin moist and supple and energy levels high. This salad tastes like a fine guacamole.

3	Roma tomatoes, diced	2	tablespoons cilantro, chopped
1½	cups cucumbers peeled with seeds removed (sliced)	1	clove garlic
		1	tablespoon liquid hot pepper sauce
½	cup radishes, sliced thin		
12	ounces romaine lettuce	1½	tablespoons lemon juice
½	avocado	3	tablespoons olive oil

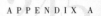
Prepare the vegetables ahead of time by washing, peeling, seeding, and cutting. Tear the Romaine lettuce into bite-sized pieces. In a bowl, mix together the avocado, cilantro, garlic, hot pepper sauce, lemon juice, and olive oil until creamy. In a larger serving bowl, combine the lettuce, tomatoes, cucumbers, and radishes. Add the desired amount of dressing and mix. Serve at once.

Black Bean Chili

Serves 10
Prep time: 20 minutes
Cook time: 1½ hours

This simple chili recipe was one of the favorites of our test group. Prepare it when you have a little time to spend in the kitchen, then freeze it in serving-size containers for a quick meal on the run. It will hold in the refrigerator for up to four days.

2	cups black beans, dried	¼	cup sun-dried tomatoes, in ¼-inch slices
4	cups water		
1	tablespoon olive oil	2	cups fat-free chicken broth
1	tablespoon garlic, chopped	2	tablespoons chili powder
½	cup carrots, peeled and diced into ¼-inch pieces	2	teaspoons cayenne pepper
		1½	tablespoons hot pepper sauce (Durkee's)
½	cup onions, peeled and diced into ¼-inch pieces		
		1	pound boneless chicken breasts, cut into ½-inch pieces
½	cup celery, diced into ¼-inch pieces		
½	cup red bell peppers, seeded and diced	¼	cup green onions, chopped
		1	cup tomatoes, diced

Soak beans overnight in water. The next day, drain them and put into a pot with enough water to cover by one inch. Simmer gently until tender (approximately 1 hour). Drain and set aside for later use. In a large pot, heat ½ tablespoon olive oil and sauté garlic for three minutes over medium heat, stirring constantly. Add carrots, onions, celery, and peppers. Cook for fifteen minutes. Add cooked black beans, sun-dried tomatoes, and chicken broth. Lower heat and cover pot with a lid. Let simmer for twenty minutes. Remove the lid and add chili powder, cayenne, and pepper sauce. Simmer twenty more minutes.

In a sauté pan, heat ½ tablespoon of olive oil and sauté chicken until done (approximately fifteen minutes). Add to chili along with the green onions, diced tomatoes, and salt and pepper to taste. Let simmer five more minutes and serve.

Meal-in-a-Flash Prep Plan
Cut up vegetables in the morning. Cook beans up to two days in advance (just keep covered in the refrigerator). You may also use canned black beans (6 cups canned), but this will increase the salt quite a bit. While beans cook, chop veggies and cut up and sauté chicken.

Black Bean Soup

Serves 10
Prep time: 25 minutes
Cook time: 3 hours

I call this a "comfort food"—the kind of soup you can enjoy on a cool wintery evening or heated just slightly for a quick meal on the run. You'll want to double the recipe and store the extra in the freezer. Heats up beautifully in the microwave for lunch.

1	pound black beans, dried (or 6 cups canned)	¼	teaspoon ground cloves
		¼	teaspoon ground allspice
1½	tablespoons olive oil	1½	cups low-sodium chicken stock
1	cup onions, chopped		
2	carrots, chopped	2	tablespoons sherry
2	stalks celery, diced	8	ounces broiled chicken breast, shredded
3	cloves garlic, minced		
2	dried bay leaves	1	tablespoon butter
1	teaspoon dried basil	1	onion, quartered and sliced
½	teaspoon dried thyme	3	tablespoons parsley

Rinse and sort the beans, discarding withered or discolored ones. Soak overnight in plenty of water. The next morning, drain the beans and rinse them again. Place in a large soup pot or Dutch oven with fresh water in three-to-one ratio, approximately. Bring to a boil, cover, and simmer on low heat for 1 hour.

Add the oil, chopped onion, carrots, celery, garlic, and the herbs and spices. Simmer for another 1 to 1½ hours or until the beans are soft. Drain off water. Add chicken stock.

With slotted spoon, scoop out 1½ cups of the beans, avoiding the other vegetables. Set aside. Discard the bay leaves. In a food processor or blender, puree the soup. Return the puree to the soup pot along with the reserved beans.

Add the sherry and chicken and season to taste with salt and pepper. Return to low heat.

In a small skillet, heat the butter until it foams. Add the sliced onion and sauté over low heat until golden brown. *Note:* The deeper brown you get the onion, the sweeter it will become. Stir the sautéed onion into the soup. Simmer for five more minutes. Garnish with chopped parsley.

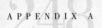

Meal-in-a-Flash Prep Plan
The soup may be prepared ahead of time and stored in the refrigerator for a few days. May also be frozen.

Baked Potato Without Fat

Serves 4

Well, this baked potato *does* contain a little butter, so it isn't totally without fat. But a little bit of butter is better than margarine! You'll never believe the great taste you get without all the fat. Makes eating a low-fat potato seem almost sinful.

4	medium russet potatoes, washed
4	tablespoons green onions, chopped
4	teaspoons paprika
2	tablespoons butter

Wash potatoes carefully. Prick holes in skin with a fork. Microwave for approximately eight minutes or bake in a 350-degree oven for forty-five minutes. Remove from oven, cut in half, fluff it up a little, and top with the rest of the ingredients.

Apple Cider Chicken

Serves 4

Prep time: 5 minutes

Cook time: 15 minutes

Reducing the apple cider/butter combination produces a flavorful sauce that delightfully enhances the flavors of the chicken breast. This recipe is simple: one that the whole family will enjoy. Be sure to make plenty for leftovers!

¾	tablespoon olive oil	½	apple, peeled, seeded, and diced
1	clove garlic, chopped		
16	ounces boneless chicken breasts, cut into 4 pieces and pounded until flattened	¾	cup apple cider or juice (unsweetened)
		1½	tablespoons butter

Heat olive oil in a sauté pan over medium-high heat and add garlic. Cook until translucent. Add chicken breasts. Cook on first side until white shows halfway up the breast (approximately four to five minutes). Flip chicken over and cook another two minutes. Add apple and sauté two minutes. Add apple cider and reduce the liquid by half. Mix in butter. Salt and pepper to taste.

Remove chicken breast and place on plate, then pour sauce and apples over the top.

Meal-in-a-Flash Prep Plan

Pound the chicken breasts in the morning or the day before. Wrap them tightly and refrigerate. You can also peel and dice the apple and put it in 1 cup of water with 1 tsp. of lemon juice. It will keep for up to two days in the refrigerator.

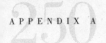

Chicken and Brown Rice Casserole

Serves 4
Prep time: 20 minutes
Cook time: 1 hour, 15 minutes

This is a simple casserole that's rich and satisfying! You can put it together in the morning before work and heat it up in the evening for a quick dinner.

1½ pounds chicken breasts, skinless	*1 egg*
2 cups cooked brown rice	*1 egg white*
½ pound broccoli, chopped	*½ teaspoon cayenne pepper*
¾ cup cheddar goat cheese, grated	*2 tablespoons basil, chopped*

Cook chicken in the oven at 350 degrees for fifteen minutes, then cool and shred. Mix all ingredients together with salt and pepper to taste, and pour into an 8-inch casserole pan. Bake at 350 degrees for forty-five minutes; remove from oven and serve.

Meal-in-a-Flash Prep Plan
Brown rice can be cooked up to two days in advance. Plan another meal with brown rice and just cook some extra for the casserole at the same time.

Chicken can be cooked up to two days in advance and kept in the refrigerator, covered tightly.

While rice is cooking, cook chicken and shred, chop broccoli, grate goat cheese, and chop basil.

Note: If you are allergic to dairy products, you may use soy cheese or other cheeses in place of goat cheese.

Chicken Tacos

Serves 4

Your kids will love this taco dish! Let them assemble their own at the table. Your family won't know they're eating "diet food!"

1	pound ground chicken		oil for frying tortillas
1	tablespoon olive oil	8	six-inch corn tortillas
1	tablespoon chili powder	2	cups lettuce, chopped
1½	cups vegetarian refried beans (canned or reconstituted)	2	ripe tomatoes, chopped

Brown chicken in olive oil just until done. Add chili powder and beans; cook until heated all the way through (approximately 5 minutes).

Heat the oil in a frying pan to very hot. Slide the tortillas into the oil, one by one, and quickly heat them, first on one side, then on the other. Press each one between two thicknesses of paper towels to absorb the extra oil.

Serve the chicken/bean mixture in taco shells with lettuce and tomatoes on top.

Meal-in-a-Flash Prep Plan
This taco mixture can be made up to three days in advance and kept in the refrigerator covered. Fry the tortillas just before serving.

Note: If you can't find ground chicken in your local market, just put boneless chicken breast in your food processor and pulse to the consistency you want.

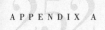

Chicken Caesar Salad

Serves 4
Prep time: 15 minutes
Cook time: 15 minutes

Main entrée salads are an excellent way to get your daily requirement of green vegetables and provide your protein requirement as well. This is a delicious Caesar salad recipe that transports to work easily. Keep it in the refrigerator at work and toss the dressing into the greens just before you enjoy it!

1	egg yolk	½	tablespoon Worcestershire sauce
½	tablespoon garlic, chopped		
½	lemon, juiced	½	cup olive oil
2	teaspoons Dijon mustard	1	pound romaine lettuce
2	anchovy fillets, or 1 tablespoon anchovy paste	1	pound chicken breasts, grilled or baked

Place the egg yolk, garlic, lemon juice, mustard, anchovies, and Worcestershire sauce in a food processor or blender and process for two minutes. Slowly drizzle in all the olive oil while the machine continues to run. Pour desired amount of dressing over romaine and toss. Slice the chicken into thin strips and place on top of salad or toss right into it.

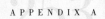

Meal-in-a-Flash Prep Plan

Lettuce can be cut and washed in advance. Wrap in a moist paper towel and place in a food storage bag and store in the refrigerator. Chicken can be cooked up to two days in advance. You can make the dressing in larger batches; it will hold in the refrigerator up to a week.

Chinese Chicken Salad

Serves 4

Prep time: 20 minutes

Cook time: 20 minutes

We served this main entrée salad to our test group at our very first meeting. Everyone was delighted with the taste and how satisfied they felt—a complete meal in a bowl!

1 tablespoon sherry vinegar*	*2 stalks celery, sliced on the diagonal in ½-inch pieces*
½ tablespoon hoisin sauce*	
½ tablespoon soy sauce	*1 cup red bell pepper, seeded and julienned*
1½ tablespoons olive oil	
1½ tablespoon sesame oil	*½ pound snow peas, cleaned and blanched*
10 ounces boneless chicken breasts	
	1 pound mixed lettuce or mesclun mix*
1 raw carrot, peeled and julienned	
	1 teaspoon sesame seeds, toasted

*See Appendix B for more information about this product.

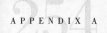

Dressing

Whisk together vinegar, hoisin sauce, and soy sauce. Slowly drizzle in the oils while continuing to whisk. When the ingredients are well blended, the dressing is done.

Chicken

Bake the chicken breasts in the oven at 350 degrees for approximately twenty minutes or until white all the way through. For extra flavor, put a little dressing on the breasts before you put them into the oven. When the chicken is done, remove it from the oven and let it cool. Shred it with your fingers.

Mixing the Salad

Mix together all vegetables and lettuce. Add shredded chicken. Add the dressing to taste and toss to coat.

Meal-in-a-Flash Prep Plan

Prepare veggies in advance and keep in refrigerator for up to a week. Salad dressing will hold mixed for up to two weeks refrigerated. Cook chicken while preparing vegetables.

255

Chicken Enchilada Casserole

Serves 4
Prep time: 15 minutes
Cook time: 60 minutes

Don't you just love casseroles? They're so easy to assemble and serve, and the whole family enjoys them. This beautiful casserole freezes well for a quick meal on the run.

1	pound chicken breasts	⅓	cup canned tomatoes, diced
1¾	cups enchilada sauce*	2	cups cheddar goat cheese, grated
8	six-inch corn tortillas		
1	cup canned green chilies		

Bake chicken in a 350-degree oven for fifteen minutes, then shred or chop. Heat the enchilada sauce until it is just warm. Use a four-inch casserole dish to layer, lasagna-style, the corn tortillas dipped in the enchilada sauce with a layer of chicken, a layer of chilies, a layer of tomatoes, and a layer of cheese.

Repeat the process two more times, pouring any remaining sauce over the top. Bake at 350 for forty-five minutes. Remove from the oven and serve.

Meal-in-a-Flash Prep Plan

Chicken can be cooked two days ahead and kept refrigerated. Casserole freezes great! ***Note:*** If you are allergic to dairy products, you may use soy cheese or other cheeses in the place of goat cheese.

---

*Found in ethnic section of grocery store.

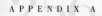
Chicken and Mushroom Casserole

Serves 4
Prep time: 10 minutes
Cook time: 45 minutes

⅓	pound mushrooms, sliced	6	ounces cheddar goat cheese, grated
1	chicken breast, cooked and shredded	½	tablespoon spelt flour*
⅓	cup frozen broccoli, thawed and chopped	⅓	cup half & half

Arrange sliced mushrooms, chicken, broccoli, and goat cheese in layers in a casserole. Blend together a pinch of salt and pepper, flour, and half & half. Pour over the layers.

Meal-in-a-Flash Prep Plan
Chicken can be cooked up to two days ahead and kept in the refrigerator. Mushrooms can be sliced in the morning. ***Note:*** If you are allergic to dairy products, you may substitute soy milk in this recipe. You may use soy cheese or other cheeses in place of goat cheese.

---

*See Appendix B for more information about this product.

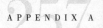
Baked Snapper with Spicy Black Beans

Serves 4

Prep time: 15 minutes

Cook time: 20 minutes

2	*tablespoons butter*	1⅓	*teaspoons garlic, chopped fine*
¾	*teaspoon lemon juice*	1⅓	*teaspoons cayenne pepper*
1¼	*teaspoons fresh thyme, chopped*	3	*teaspoons chili powder*
1	*pound snapper, bones removed*	3	*tablespoons sun-dried tomatoes, julienned*
1⅓	*teaspoons olive oil*	2	*tablespoons cilantro, chopped*
3	*tablespoons onions, diced fine*	4	*cups black beans, cooked or canned*

Mix together butter, lemon juice, and thyme. Place the snapper in a baking dish and top with butter mixture. Bake in a 350-degree oven until done (approximately fifteen minutes).

Heat the olive oil in a saucepan. Add the onions and garlic and cook for three minutes. Add remaining ingredients and cook until beans are heated through (approximately fifteen minutes). Ladle the beans onto plates and arrange snapper on top. Serve immediately.

Meal-in-a-Flash Prep Plan

Prepare the beans while snapper is cooking.

Cider-Poached Cod with Caramelized Onions

Serves 4

This creamy yet tangy dish is sure to make you feel warm on a wintry day. Easy to prepare, too!

2	teaspoons olive oil
1½	cup onions, sliced thin
20	ounces fresh cod fillet, cut in half
¾	cup apple cider, unsweetened
1	teaspoon lemon juice
2	teaspoons butter

Heat olive oil in a sauté pan. Add onions. Cook over medium heat, stirring constantly until dark brown in color (the onions will taste sweeter). Remove from heat and add the cod. Pour in apple cider. Cover the pan and put it in a 450-degree oven for approximately fifteen minutes (cooking time will depend on the thickness of the fish).

Remove the fish and onions and arrange on serving plates. Place the pan with remaining liquid on medium heat and add lemon juice. Reduce liquid by one quarter and add butter. Stir in butter completely and pour sauce over the fish.

Note: Onions can be cooked up to a week in advance if kept refrigerated.

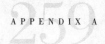

Cioppino

Serves 6
Prep time: 20 minutes
Cook time: 45 minutes

Cioppino (pronounced Choe-PEA-no) is a red seafood stew, full of vegetables and a variety of foods from the sea. The diverse flavors and textures blend together to make a warming, soothing, filling dish you may want to serve to special guests.

1	tablespoon olive oil	1½	pounds cod, cut into bite-sized pieces
3	celery stalks, chopped		
1	cup fennel, chopped fine	¼	pound crab
2	carrots, peeled and chopped	½	pound bay shrimp
1	onion, peeled and chopped	½	tablespoon liquid hot pepper sauce (Durkee's)
2	cups clam juice		
2	cups canned tomatoes, chopped	1	teaspoon thyme

Heat olive oil in a pan and add celery, fennel, carrots, and onion. Cook until tender. Add clam juice and tomatoes. Bring to a boil. Add cod, crab, shrimp, hot sauce, and thyme. Let simmer for half an hour. Season with salt and pepper and serve.

Meal-in-a-Flash Prep Plan
This fisherman's stew can be prepared in the morning. Just let it simmer for fifteen minutes before refrigerating for the day. Finish cooking in the evening. It may also be frozen and reheated. Vegetables can be chopped in the food processor.

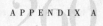

Crab Cakes

Serves 4
Prep time: 15 minutes
Cook time: 15 minutes

And you thought only gourmet cooks make crab cakes! These cakes are so simple, you'll want to make them often. And so delicious, guests will beg for the recipe. Don't be afraid to substitute imitation crab for the real thing. Most people can't tell the difference in this recipe.

18	ounces crab meat (or imitation crab)	1	lemon, juiced
		½	teaspoon wasabi powder*
1	cucumber, peeled and diced, seeds removed	¼	teaspoon cayenne pepper
		8	tablespoons dry potato flakes
2	eggs	2	tablespoons olive oil
2	stalks celery, diced		

Mix all ingredients together, except 1 tablespoon potato flakes and olive oil. Mixture should hold together. If mixture seems too wet, add more potato flakes. Shape into six patties. Lightly dust with remaining potato flakes. Heat olive oil in a sauté pan over medium heat. Place crab cakes in the pan carefully. Cook on one side until brown (approximately four minutes). Flip over and cook another four to five minutes. Remove from pan and serve with lemon caper sauce.

---

*See Appendix B for more information about this product.

Meal-in-a-Flash Prep Plan

Crab mixture can be made ahead of time and left refrigerated for up to two days. It will become wet the longer it sits, so you might need to add more potato flakes to it before making patties. Remember not to dust with potato flakes until right before cooking or the cakes will be soggy.

Note: If your store doesn't carry wasabi powder, you may leave it out.

Lemon Caper Sauce

Serves 4

This lovely sauce goes well with the crab cakes.

1½ tablespoons parsley, chopped fine	2 teaspoons vinegar
1 tablespoon onion, finely diced	2 tablespoons lemon juice
	½ cup low-fat mayonnaise
1¼ teaspoon Dijon mustard	1 tablespoon capers

Place the parsley, onion, mustard, vinegar, and lemon juice in a bowl and mix together. Mix in the mayonnaise and capers. Serve right away or refrigerate. This sauce will keep up to three days in the refrigerator.

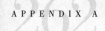

Curried Seafood Stew

Serves 4
Prep time: 20 minutes
Cook time: 15 minutes

Don't be intimidated by the ingredients in this recipe. It is well worth the trouble to locate these specialty items and keep them on hand. You'll be making this savory stew often!

1	tablespoon olive oil	1	cup coconut milk*
1	pound prawns, peeled and deveined	2	cups chicken broth
½	cup celery, diced into ½-inch pieces	1	tablespoon curry paste*
		1	teaspoon fish sauce*
½	cup onions, diced into ½-inch pieces	½	pound crab meat (or imitation crab)
2	carrots, diced into ½-inch pieces	12	ounces cod, in 1½-inch pieces

Heat olive oil over medium high heat in a pot and add prawns. Cook until pink in color (approximately three minutes). Remove prawns and add vegetables, then cook another three minutes. Add coconut milk, chicken broth, curry paste, fish sauce, and crab meat, and bring to a boil. Let simmer for ten minutes. Add cod and prawns back into stew and let simmer five more minutes. Remove from heat and serve over rice.

Note: You can find coconut milk, curry paste, and fish sauce in the specialty section of the grocery store. If you can't find curry

---

*See Appendix B for more information about this product.

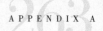

paste, substitute curry powder. And if you can't find fish sauce, it's okay to leave it out.

Lemon Pepper Halibut

Serves 4
Prep time: 10 minutes
Cook time: 20 minutes

A light, zesty version of halibut. You won't need lemon wedges with this dish. When possible, use fresh halibut. If it is not available fresh, you may substitute any other white, mild-flavored fish.

2	*lemons, zested*	20	*ounces halibut fillets*
1	*teaspoon lemon pepper*	⅓	*cup rice wine (sake)*
3	*sprigs fresh thyme, chopped*	2	*teaspoons butter*
	Dash olive oil		

Zest the lemons by grating the skin on the fine side of your food grater. Mix together the lemon zest, lemon pepper, and thyme. Smear over fish along with a dash of olive oil. Let marinate for at least one hour (the longer the better). Place the fish in a pan and put into a 400-degree oven for approximately fifteen minutes (cooking time will differ, according to thickness of fish).

Remove the pan from the oven and place the fish on a plate. Place pan over medium heat and deglaze with sake and the juice of half of one lemon. Let liquid reduce by half and mix in butter. Pour sauce over the halibut and serve.

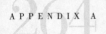

Stuffed Fillet of Sole

Serves 4
Prep time: 15 minutes
Cook time: 20 minutes

You may substitute any mild-flavored fish for the sole if it is unavailable. Very pretty when served on the plate, and it tastes wonderful as well!

24	ounces sole	½	teaspoon garlic, chopped
1	tablespoon olive oil	½	tablespoon parsley, chopped
2	tablespoons red bell peppers, diced small	2	teaspoons lemon juice
2	tablespoons celery, diced small	¾	cup white wine
2	tablespoons carrots, diced small	2	tablespoons butter
		½	teaspoon paprika

Heat the olive oil in a sauté pan over medium heat and sauté the bell peppers, celery, carrots, and garlic for five minutes. Remove the pan from heat and add parsley, cilantro, and lemon juice. Salt and pepper to taste. Portion out the sole into six 4-oz. portions and lay them out with the back side up.

Divide the vegetable mixture among the six fillets and place in the middle of each. Roll up the fillets so the stuffing is in the inside. Place in a baking dish, pour wine into the bottom of the baking dish, and sprinkle each fillet with a little paprika.

Bake at 400 degrees for twelve to fifteen minutes or until the fish flakes. Remove from heat. Remove the fish from the pan and mix butter into whatever liquid remains. Pour over the fish and serve immediately.

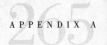

Meal-in-a-Flash Prep Plan

You can cut up the vegetables ahead of time and keep in the refrigerator or sauté them ahead of time and keep in the refrigerator for up to two days. Vegetables can also be chopped with food processor.

Seasoned Beef in Corn Tortillas

Serves 6
Prep time: 20 minutes
Cook time: 2 hours, 15 minutes

This Mexican-style beef dish takes a little while to prepare, so plan ahead. Cook the stew meat the evening before you plan to serve it. This is another recipe your kids (and your friends) will enjoy. Very savory, and the beef is very tender.

2	*pounds beef stew meat, all fat trimmed off*	1	*teaspoon salt*
1½	*cups water*	1	*teaspoon ground cumin*
2	*cloves garlic, minced*	⅛	*teaspoon pepper*
2	*tablespoons chili powder*	12	*ten-inch corn tortillas*
1	*tablespoon vinegar*	2	*cups shredded romaine lettuce*
2	*teaspoons dried oregano, crushed*		

In medium saucepan, combine meat, water, garlic, chili powder, vinegar, oregano, salt, cumin, and pepper. Bring to boil. Cover, reduce heat, and simmer about two hours or until meat is very tender. Uncover and boil rapidly about fifteen minutes or until water has almost evaporated. Watch closely and stir near end of cooking time so meat doesn't stick. Remove from heat. Using two forks, finely shred meat.

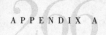

Stack tortillas in foil; heat in 340-degree oven for fifteen minutes. Spoon about ¼ cup meat mixture and a handful of the shredded lettuce onto each tortilla, near one edge. Fold edge nearest filling up and over filling just until mixture is covered. Fold in the two sides envelope fashion, then roll up. Fasten with wooden pick if needed.

Garnish with lettuce. One serving equals two "chimi-changas."

Itsa Meatball

Serves 6
Prep time: 15 minutes
Cook time: 1 hour

It's a quick trip to Italy with our variation of this traditional recipe for Italian-style meatballs. Easy to prepare in advance, and the kids will love the tasty meatballs on top of their favorite pasta.

⅓	cup whole goat or soy milk	1	tablespoon vegetable oil
½	cup oatmeal	½	teaspoon salt
1	pound extra-lean ground beef	4	ten-ounce cans tomato sauce
1	tablespoon onion, finely chopped	3	cloves garlic, diced
		½	teaspoon dried oregano
1	tablespoon parsley, chopped	½	teaspoon dried parsley
1	egg	½	teaspoon dried basil
3	tablespoons Parmesan cheese, finely grated	½	pound corn pasta

Heat the milk in a small saucepan and add the oatmeal. Stir and let sit while you prepare the rest of the ingredients. In a mixing

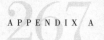

bowl, combine the chopped meat, onion, parsley, egg, Parmesan cheese, oil, the oatmeal/milk mixture, and salt. Mix everything thoroughly but gently. (Mixes better by hand!)

Without squeezing, shape the mixture into small round balls, about one inch in diameter. Broil the meatballs on each side until lightly browned, turning several times.

Meanwhile, prepare the tomato sauce by combining the sauce with the garlic and herbs (oregano, parsley, basil) and let it simmer gently while preparing the meatballs.

When the meatballs have browned, add to the tomato sauce and slowly simmer, covered, for another forty-five minutes or until the meatballs are cooked thoroughly. Make sure the sauce does not stick.

Bring a pot of water to a boil and add the corn pasta. Simmer gently for ten minutes or until tender. Serve with the meatballs and sauce.

Meal-in-a-Flash Prep Plan
The meatballs and sauce can be made ahead of time and stored in the refrigerator. Thirty minutes before mealtime, heat the sauce gently. Be careful not to scorch. Stir carefully so you don't break the meatballs. Meanwhile, fix the pasta and serve dinner!

Mock Filet Mignon

Serves 6
Prep time: 15 minutes
Cook time: 15–20 minutes

This was another favorite in our test groups. The comment I frequently heard was: "My kids love it and want me to serve it again!"

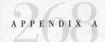

1½	pounds lean ground beef	1½	teaspoons salt
2	cups cooked rice	¼	teaspoon ground pepper
1	cup onion, minced	6	slices turkey bacon
1	teaspoon garlic, minced		
2	tablespoons Worcestershire sauce		

Preheat oven to 450 degrees. Combine ground beef with rice, onion, garlic, Worcestershire sauce, salt, and pepper. Blend well; shape into six round patties (about one inch thick).

Wrap a strip of turkey bacon around each patty; fasten with a wooden pick. Place in an ungreased shallow baking pan. Bake fifteen minutes or until bacon is cooked and beef patties are done as desired. Remove picks before serving. Be sure to drain off as much fat as possible.

Meal-in-a-Flash Prep Plan
Combine the ingredients, form patties, and wrap with bacon in the morning. Cover tightly and refrigerate.

Salisbury Steak

Serves 6
Prep time: 10 minutes
Cook time: 20 minutes

A homey dish that will bring back memories of your childhood, but this is a lower fat version than the one we grew up with. You may add fresh mushrooms to the gravy if you prefer!

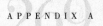
1½	pounds extra-lean ground beef		Olive oil
1	teaspoon salt	2	tablespoons spelt* or oat flour
¼	teaspoon pepper	1	4-ounce can sliced mushrooms (or fresh)
1	teaspoon Worcestershire sauce	1	cup fat-free beef broth
1	tablespoon minced onion		

Mix ground beef with seasonings and onion and shape into patties. Brown in small amount of olive oil in a skillet. Cook to desired doneness. Remove to a hot platter.

Pour off all but two tablespoons of fat. Blend in the flour. Add undrained mushrooms and beef broth and let the gravy thicken. Spoon over patties and serve.

Pan-Fried Soba Noodles

Serves 4
Prep time: 10 minutes
Cook time: 10 minutes

Lightly seasoned noodles with a little bit of crispness. They're also good served cold.

2	teaspoons sesame oil	1	teaspoon soy sauce
2	teaspoons olive oil	4	tablespoons green onions, sliced thin
12	ounces cooked Japanese Soba noodles*	1	tablespoon sesame seeds

*See Appendix B for more information about this product.

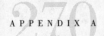

Heat oils in a medium-sized sauté pan or wok over medium heat. Add noodles and cook for four minutes. Add soy sauce, green onions, and sesame seeds. Cook to heat through. Remove from heat and serve.

Pasta Primavera and Chicken with Red Sauce

Serves 4
Prep time: 25 minutes
Cook time: 1 hour

This recipe looks daunting—so many ingredients! You will want to prepare this lovely meal when you have had a little time to prepare the ingredients in advance. Especially good as a "company meal."

1½	tablespoons olive oil	1	summer squash, sliced on angle
¾	tablespoon garlic, chopped		
4	cups canned tomatoes, chopped	⅛	pound snow peas, picked and stemmed
½	cup fresh basil, chopped	½	cup mushrooms, sliced
½	red bell pepper, roasted	1	pound chicken breasts, cut into bite-sized pieces
1½	carrots, peeled and sliced on angle		
1	red bell pepper, seeded and julienned	6	ounces corn pasta,* dry

---

*See Appendix B for more information about this product.

Preparing the Red Sauce

Heat 1 tablespoon olive oil and add 1 tablespoon garlic. Cook until translucent. Add tomatoes, basil, and roasted bell pepper. Simmer for one hour. Puree sauce in a food processor or blender, and season with salt and pepper.

Preparing the Primavera

Heat 1 tablespoon olive oil in sauté pan. Add 1 teaspoon garlic and cook until translucent. Add carrots and bell pepper. Cook until halfway done. Add the rest of the vegetables and cook until tender (two to three minutes). Add cooked vegetables to red sauce.

Preparing the Chicken

Heat ½ tablespoon olive oil in the same pan used for the vegetables. Add chicken and sauté until done. Add to red sauce and vegetables.

Preparing the Pasta

Bring a large pot of water to a boil with a little salt added. Add pasta and stir. Cook pasta until done (about ten minutes). Continue to stir pasta occasionally so it doesn't stick together. Drain pasta. Either mix together with the vegetables and sauce, or arrange the pasta on a plate and top with the red sauce.

Meal-in-a-Flash Prep Plan

Prepare the red sauce and place in refrigerator. Cut up and prepare the vegetables and place in a food storage bag in the refrigerator. Cut up the chicken and wrap tightly. Don't cook the vegetables or chicken in advance; it will make them mushy. Vegetables need to be crisp!

While the red sauce cooks you can prepare and cook vegetables along with the chicken. Cook the pasta about ten minutes before your sauce is done.

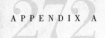
Pasta Side Dish

Serves 4
Prep time: 5 minutes
Cook time: 10 minutes

Corn pasta is an excellent substitute for wheat pasta. This is a tasty side dish that goes well with the Apple Cider Chicken.

6	ounces corn pasta*	2	tablespoons fresh parsley, chopped
2	tablespoons olive oil		
2	teaspoons garlic, chopped		

Cook pasta in boiling water until al dente (still firm but not crunchy). Heat olive oil in a sauté pan over medium heat and add garlic, cooking for three minutes. Toss in pasta and parsley. Add salt and pepper to taste, and serve.

Roasted Chicken Breast

Serves 4
Prep time: 5 minutes
Cook time: 20 minutes

2	whole skinless, boneless chicken breasts, split	¼	teaspoon salt
2	tablespoons olive oil	¼	teaspoon pepper

---

*See Appendix B for more information about this product.

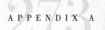

Rinse chicken breasts and pat dry. Rub each piece with olive oil. Sprinkle with salt and pepper. Place chicken on a rack in preheated oven. Roast at 400 degrees for twenty minutes or until juices run clear. Be careful not to overcook or it will be dry and stringy.

Roasted Chicken with Mushroom Gravy

Serves 4
Prep time: 10–15 minutes
Cook time: 1 hour

Lift your roasted chicken to new heights with this delicious mushroom gravy. The aroma of the garlic will waft through your house and bring your whole family down for dinner. This dish can be served with or without the gravy.

1	3-pound roasting chicken	4	tablespoons spelt* or oat flour
2	lemons		
10	cloves garlic, peeled and left whole	1	cup low-sodium chicken stock
2	sprigs fresh rosemary	1	tablespoon fresh sage, chopped
¼	teaspoon pepper		
¼	teaspoon salt	1	cup mushrooms, sliced
2	tablespoons butter		

Remove the giblets from inside the chicken and place the chicken in a roasting pan. Fill the inside of the chicken with the lemons (cut in half), garlic, and rosemary. Lightly sprinkle the salt and pepper over the chicken. Bake in the oven at 350 de-

*See Appendix B for more information about this product.

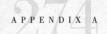

grees for one hour. Remove and serve. Make gravy while chicken cooks.

Gravy Directions

Melt butter in a sauté pan over medium heat. Whisk in the flour and cook for two minutes. Add the chicken stock, sage, and mushrooms. Bring to a boil while stirring, then simmer slowly for fifteen minutes.

Meal-in-a-Flash Prep Time

The garlic can be peeled days in advance and kept refrigerated. The chicken can be stuffed in the morning.

Roasted Turkey Breast

Serves 4

Prep time: 5 minutes

Cook time: 1 hour

If you think turkey breast is dry and flavorless, think again! This turkey breast is moist and tender, and the flavor is terrific. When possible, purchase organic, fresh turkey breast for a better flavor.

1	16-ounce turkey breast	¼	teaspoon salt
3	cloves garlic, minced	¼	teaspoon pepper
2	sprigs fresh rosemary, finely chopped		

Place the turkey in a roasting pan. Mix the garlic and rosemary together and rub over the turkey. Salt and pepper to taste. Bake uncovered in the oven at 350 degrees for one hour or until the turkey is cooked through. Be careful not to overcook or the turkey will be dry.

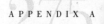

Roasted Asparagus

Serves 4
Prep time: 5 minutes
Cook time: 10 minutes

This is our family's favorite asparagus recipe—it has a light roasted flavor that will make you remember why you love asparagus.

1	*pound asparagus, bottoms trimmed*
2	*tablespoons olive oil*
	Salt and pepper to taste

Place the washed asparagus on a cookie sheet and brush with olive oil. Sprinkle with salt and pepper. Place the asparagus in a 350-degree oven for 10 minutes or until it is tender to the touch. Remove from the oven and serve.

Note: This can be cooked up to two days in advance and refrigerated.

Roasted Vegetables

Serves 4
Prep time: 15 minutes
Cook time: 25 minutes

Even kids like vegetables prepared this way. If you like a little extra flavor, brown the vegetables slightly under the broiler just before serving.

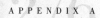
1	cup onions	10	cloves garlic, peeled
1	cup carrots, peeled	2	sprigs rosemary
1	cup celery	½	teaspoon salt
1	cup red bell pepper	½	teaspoon black pepper
1	cup zucchini	1	yellow potato
2	tablespoons olive oil		

Cut all vegetables into 1-inch pieces. Mix all the ingredients together and place in a roasting pan uncovered. Put into a 350-degree oven for approximately 25 minutes or until the vegetables are tender. Remove and serve.

Meal-in-a-Flash Prep Time
Vegetables can be cut up to a week in advance and kept tightly wrapped in the refrigerator. They can also be roasted in advance and reheated just before serving.

Fresh Veggies

Serves 4

2	raw carrots, peeled and cut into sticks	1	cup jicama,* peeled and cut into sticks
4	stalks raw celery, cut into sticks	1	raw tomato, quartered
1	cup sliced mushrooms	½	cup fat-free Ranch dressing for dipping

---

*See Appendix B for more information about this product.

Prepare these tasty vegetables ahead of time! They will easily store in a bowl of water for several days. Enjoy them with a small amount of Ranch dressing for dipping.

Sautéed Broccoli

Serves 4

A nice way to add greens to your diet!

1½ pounds broccoli flowers
2   tablespoons butter
    Salt and pepper to taste

Melt butter in a sauté pan. Add broccoli and cook for five to seven minutes. Season to taste and serve.

Sautéed Green and Yellow Beans

Serves 4

½ pound raw green beans,   ¾ tablespoon butter
     stemmed   1   teaspoon garlic, chopped
½ pound yellow beans,   Salt and pepper to taste
     stemmed

Add beans to boiling water and cook for five minutes. Drain. Heat butter and garlic in a sauté pan for one minute. Add the beans and saute for three minutes. Season and serve.

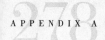

Meal-in-a-Flash Prep Plan

Stem the beans in the morning. They can even be blanched, but make sure to cool them completely. Sauté cooked beans for five minutes so they will be warm all the way through.

Sautéed Zucchini

Serves 4

Turns this otherwise bland vegetable into a more tasty version! Especially good for that bountiful end-of-summer crop!

---

4   cups zucchini, sliced
1   clove garlic, chopped
2   tablespoons olive oil

Heat olive oil in a sauté pan. Add garlic and squash. Cook until tender.

Thai Vegetables with Chicken and Rice

Serves 4
Prep time: 20 minutes
Cook time: 55 minutes

This is one of my all-time favorite recipes. The aroma will bring your neighbors to your door! You'll want to serve this recipe to both guests and family. Yes, it takes a little time to prepare, but it's worth every moment!

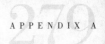

1	red bell pepper, seeded and sliced	⅛	teaspoon fish sauce*
1	carrot, peeled and sliced	¾	tablespoon hot chili paste*
1	onion, peeled and sliced	1	tablespoon olive oil
½	pound snow peas, stemmed	1	pound boneless chicken breasts, cut into bite-sized pieces
1	summer squash, sliced		Steamed Rice (see p. 281)
¾	cup coconut milk*		
1½	cups basic vegetable stock		

Prepare the vegetables, slicing them on the diagonal for additional flavor and visual appeal. Set aside.

In a saucepan, mix together the coconut milk, vegetable stock, fish sauce, and chili paste. Bring to a boil and reduce heat to medium. Reduce sauce by over half (takes about forty-five minutes).

In a separate pan, heat olive oil and add chicken. When chicken is ¾ cooked (about five minutes), add all the vegetables. Sauté for three minutes, stirring frequently, and add the reduced sauce. Bring sauce to a boil. Remove from heat and arrange chicken, vegetables, and sauce mixture over rice. Serve immediately.

Meal-in-a-Flash Prep Plan

In the morning or when you have a little time, prepare the sauce and slice the vegetables. Place the vegetables in a food storage bag and refrigerate. Refrigerate the sauce (can be refrigerated for up to a week).

You may also prepare the rice at this time. Reheat the rice about fifteen minutes before dinner is served. In a separate pan, sauté chicken and vegetables. Add the sauce, and finish.

*See Appendix B for more information about this product.

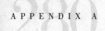
Sesame Chicken with Stir-Fried Vegetables

Serves 4

Prep time: 20 minutes

Cook time: 20 minutes

A touch of the Asian flavor we all love. This is a stir-fry recipe you'll want to prepare often.

20	ounces boneless chicken breasts, cut into one-inch pieces	1	red bell pepper, seeded and sliced thin
4	teaspoons sesame seeds	1	carrot, peeled and sliced thin
	Salt and pepper to taste	2	celery stalks, sliced thin
1	tablespoon olive oil	1	cup snow peas, stemmed
3	cups cabbage, sliced thin	4	teaspoons white wine vinegar
½	pound mushrooms, stemmed and sliced thin	4	teaspoons soy sauce
		1½	teaspoon sesame oil
		1	teaspoon ginger, grated

Coat chicken with sesame seeds and season with salt and pepper. Heat olive oil in a sauté pan to medium heat. Add chicken and cook for about five minutes. Add cabbage and cook for three minutes. Add remaining vegetables and cook for additional five minutes.

In a bowl, combine vinegar, soy sauce, sesame oil, ginger, and chili oil. Add to chicken and vegetables and cook for one minute. Remove from heat and serve.

Meal-in-a-Flash Prep Plan
Prepare the vegetables up to three days in advance.

Steamed Rice

Serves 4

⅔ cup rice
1⅓ cups water

Rinse rice until water runs clear. Place in a baking dish and add water. Cover baking dish with foil and bake in a 350-degree oven for thirty minutes. Rice should be fluffy when done.

Shepherd's Pie

Serves 6
Prep time: 20 minutes
Cook time: 30 minutes

A weight-loss version of a favorite you enjoyed from your childhood. Introduce this traditional recipe to your children—they'll enjoy it as well. You won't leave the table hungry.

1½	pounds ground turkey	¼	teaspoon dried thyme
1	onion, chopped	1	cup frozen peas, thawed
2	cloves garlic, minced	1	cup frozen corn, thawed
1	stalk celery, chopped	2½	cups mashed potatoes
½	teaspoon dried parsley	½	cup cheddar goat cheese,
½	teaspoon dried oregano		grated

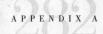

Fry the turkey with the onion, garlic, and celery in a tiny bit of olive oil just until it turns color. Add the herbs and stir to mix well. Spread the turkey mixture over the bottom of a casserole. Combine the peas and corn and spread over the turkey. Spread the potatoes like frosting over the peas and corn. Sprinkle the grated cheese over the whole mixture. Bake in a 350-degree oven for twenty minutes or until hot through and the cheese is melted.

Note: Freezes well. While potatoes boil, cook and chop everything else. If you are allergic to goat cheese, you may substitute soy cheese, but the flavor will not be as nice.

Grandma's Turkey Soup

Serves 10
Prep time: 30 minutes
Cook time: 4 hours

3	quarts water	½	teaspoon salt
5	pounds turkey legs, thighs, and wings	½	teaspoon pepper
		½	cup long-grain brown rice
1	cup chopped onion		10-ounce package frozen peas, thawed
1	cup chopped celery		
1	cup sliced carrots	2	tablespoons sage
2½	cups diced potatoes	1½	teaspoon soy sauce
	16-ounce can tomato puree		
	14-ounce can tomatoes with liquid		

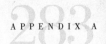

Cover and simmer turkey parts in water for three hours. Remove turkey; discard bones and skin. Shred meat; set aside. (You should have about 4 cups of meat.)

Thoroughly defat broth.* Simmer onion, celery, carrots, potatoes, tomato puree, tomatoes, and salt and pepper in stock for twenty minutes, covered, until vegetables are tender. Add rice and cook for thirty minutes. Return meat to stock.

Add peas and cook additional ten minutes or until rice is done and vegetables are tender. Season with sage and soy sauce.

Note: This soup freezes and reheats wonderfully.

Lentil Soup with Herbs

Serves 4

A lovely, hearty soup that freezes well for a quick meal later in the week when you're rushed for time.

3¾ cups water	1 teaspoon fresh oregano, chopped
½ clove garlic, chopped fine	½ teaspoon paprika
½ onion, diced fine	¼ teaspoon salt
1 carrot, chopped	1 teaspoon fresh parsley, chopped
1 stalk celery, chopped	1½ teaspoons olive oil
¾ cup dried lentils	
1½ teaspoon red miso†	
½ teaspoon fresh thyme, chopped	

---

*To defat broth: Use a defatting cup (can be purchased from a kitchen specialty shop), or allow the broth to thoroughly chill and then remove the solid fat from the top.
†See Appendix B for more information about this product.

Bring the water to a boil in a large soup kettle. Add garlic, onion, carrot, celery, lentils, and miso. Return to a boil. Add seasonings and mix well. Simmer, covered, over low heat for sixty minutes. Use a potato masher to partially puree the soup in the kettle, mashing it as much as you like. Remove from heat and stir in the parsley and the oil.

Note: Vegetable bouillon can be substituted for the miso if you wish.

Meal-in-a-Flash Prep Plan
The entire soup can be prepared ahead of time. Freezes well.

Southwestern Chili

Serves 4–6
Prep time: 15 minutes
Cook time: 1½ hours

We still get rave comments about this chili! Thick and hearty with just a touch of spices that tingle the taste buds. Double the recipe; you'll want leftovers.

1	tablespoon olive oil	4	cups red kidney beans, canned
1	onion, chopped		
1¼	pounds ground turkey	¼	cup tomato paste
4	cups canned tomatoes, chopped	2	tablespoons chili powder
			Salt and pepper to taste

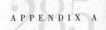
Heat olive oil in a pot and add onion. Cook until tender. Add turkey and cook until done. Add tomatoes, kidney beans, tomato paste, and chili powder. Bring to a boil, lower heat, and simmer for one hour. Add salt and pepper and serve.

Tortilla Chicken Soup

Serves 6
Prep time: 15 minutes
Cook time: ½ hour

This is not only chicken soup for the soul; it's chicken soup for the body! Lightly seasoned to wake up the taste buds. Soothing on a cold winter evening.

1	*pound chicken breasts*	4	*cups chicken stock*
2	*cups canned green chilies*	2	*cups canned tomatoes, diced*
6	*corn tortillas*	1	*tablespoon cayenne pepper*
½	*cup cheddar goat cheese (or soy cheese), grated*	¼	*cup canola oil*

Bake the chicken at 350 degrees for fifteen minutes, then cool and shred. Set aside. Cut the chilies into small pieces. Slice the tortillas into bite-sized pieces; grate the goat cheese and set aside.

In a soup pot, bring chicken stock to a boil and add chilies, tomatoes, and cayenne. Simmer for half an hour, then add chicken. Heat the oil in a sauté pan and fry the tortillas until crisp. Drain on paper towels.

Dish out soup into bowls, sprinkle tortilla pieces on top, add cheese. Serve at once.

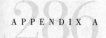

Meal-in-a-Flash Prep Plan

Chicken can be cooked up to two days in advance. Tortillas can be fried in the morning. Chicken can also be cooking while soup is simmering.

White Bean Minestrone

Serves 4
Prep time: 25 minutes
Cook time: 1 hour, 30 minutes

Bean soup is an excellent source of fiber. This is an American-ized version of an old Italian home recipe. This soup can warm you up on a cold day or provide a light supper on a warm evening.

½ cup small white beans, dry	1 stalk celery, cut in half-inch pieces
¾ cup corn pasta	¼ head cabbage, sliced thin
1 tablespoon olive oil	2 tablespoons fresh basil, chopped
4 slices turkey bacon, in quarter-inch pieces	2 cups canned tomatoes, in juice
½ clove garlic, chopped	
3 raw carrots, peeled and cut in half-inch pieces	1½ cups chicken broth
1 onion, peeled and cut in half-inch pieces	1½ cups beef broth

---

Soak beans in five cups of water overnight, then drain and add fresh water. Bring to a boil. Cook until tender (approximately forty-five minutes). Drain off water and set aside. Cook pasta and cool. Set aside.

Heat olive oil in large pot over medium heat. Add bacon and

cook until brown. Add garlic and cook for two minutes, then add the vegetables. Cook vegetables for fifteen minutes, add basil, tomatoes, and stocks. Increase heat and bring to a boil. Lower heat and simmer for thirty minutes, then add beans and simmer for another fifteen minutes.

Adjust seasonings with salt and pepper to taste, then add the cooked pasta. Simmer for five minutes and serve.

Meal-in-a-Flash Prep Plan
Beans can be cooked up to two days in advance. Just cover and refrigerate. Pasta may also be cooked two days ahead. Just coat with a little oil and refrigerate. Vegetables can be cut up ahead of time.

Wheat-Free Corn Bread

Serves 8

Remember how delicious corn bread is when you pull it, steaming, out of the oven? You simply must bake your corn bread in an iron skillet for a crisp exterior, and if you preheat the skillet, it will be even crispier. If you have any leftovers, your kids may enjoy it toasted lightly for breakfast.

1	tablespoon canola oil	¼	teaspoon salt
1	cup yellow stoneground corn-meal	1	egg
½	cup spelt* or oat flour	3	tablespoons honey
2	teaspoons baking powder	1	cup whole goat milk or soy milk

*See Appendix B for more information about this product.

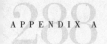
Preheat oven to 375 degrees. Rub an 8-inch baking pan or a black iron skillet with 1 teaspoon of the oil. In a bowl, sift together cornmeal, flour, baking powder, and salt. Add egg, honey, and remaining oil. Mix until smooth. Add milk and blend thoroughly. Pour into pan and place in the oven for twenty-five to thirty minutes, or until a toothpick inserted in the middle comes out clean. Remove from oven and let cool until just warm. Cut and serve.

super snack ideas!

Avocado Salad

½   ripe avocado, peeled and
        seeded
1   tablespoon olive oil
½   tablespoon lemon juice
     Other seasonings to taste

Mix together the oil, lemon juice, and seasonings, and sprinkle over the avocado half. Enjoy as a satisfying snack!

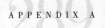
Buffalo Chicken Wings

½	cup Simple and Quick Barbecue Sauce (see page 292)	3	tablespoons butter
½	cup Liquid Hot Pepper Sauce (Durkee's)	16	chicken wings (drumettes)

In a saucepan, combine the barbecue sauce, hot sauce, and butter. Bring to a boil, then lower heat and simmer for fifteen minutes. In a baking dish, lay out wings in a single layer and brush with sauce. Place in a 350-degree oven for fifteen minutes until done. Brush once more with sauce. Use as much sauce as you want heat. (The more sauce you use, the hotter it will be.)

Chicken Pâté

1½	pounds chicken breasts, skinned and boned	1	tablespoon brandy
1	cup cream	2	tablespoons parsley
1	egg	2	tablespoons chives
1	egg white	1	tablespoon tarragon

Slice ½ pound of the chicken breast into thin strips and place to the side for assembly.

Place the remaining chicken in the food processor and puree until smooth. Slowly add the cream until incorporated, then add remaining ingredients. Spray a loaf pan with nonstick spray. Pour in half of the chicken mixture and smooth out. Lay down the thin strips of chicken and cover with remaining chicken mixture.

Place loaf pan in a bigger pan with water (water bath) and bake in a 400-degree oven for forty-five minutes. Should feel like a meat loaf when done. Remove from oven and let rest five minutes before serving. Slice and arrange decoratively on a lettuce leaf, with pickles, olives, or other accompaniments.

Sinful Deviled Eggs

8   eggs, hard-boiled and peeled
2   tablespoons low-calorie
       mayonnaise
½   teaspoon lemon juice
⅛   teaspoon paprika
     Salt to taste

Slice the eggs in half lengthwise. Carefully remove yolks. Place yolks in a bowl and smash with a fork. Mix in mayonnaise and lemon juice. Spoon back into egg halves and sprinkle with paprika.

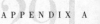
Roasted, Toasted Pumpkin Seeds

½	pound raw pumpkin seeds	*Salt to taste*
1	tablespoon olive oil	

Coat the pumpkin seeds with the olive oil, mixing carefully to distribute the oil throughout. Spread out on a baking sheet in a thin layer and bake at 350 degrees for about ten minutes or until crispy and lightly browned. Be careful not to burn. Remove from the oven and sprinkle with salt. Let cool thoroughly. Can be used on salads or eaten as a snack.

bonus recipes!

Simple and Quick Barbecued Chicken

Serves 2

½	cup Simple and Quick Barbecue Sauce (p. 292)
2	pounds skinless chicken legs

Preheat broiler. Wash the chicken legs carefully and place in a baking dish. Spoon a portion of the barbecue sauce over each leg and spread around carefully to cover lightly. Place under the broiler unit in the oven, leaving the door slightly ajar. Broil until nicely browned, turning and basting with sauce as each side browns.

Turn the oven down to 375 degrees. Close the oven door and bake just until chicken legs are done (about fifteen minutes). Remove pan, drain off any excess fat, and serve immediately.

Simple and Quick Barbecue Sauce

Serves 4

---

1 clove garlic, minced	1½ tablespoons lemon juice
⅓ cup catsup, reduced calorie, low salt	½ teaspoon pepper
	2 tablespoons honey
3 tablespoons brown sugar, un-packed	1 tablespoon liquid hot pepper sauce (Durkee's)
1½ tablespoons red wine vinegar	
1 cup black bean sauce*	

Place all ingredients in a small pan and simmer for thirty minutes.

Meal-in-a-Flash Prep Plan
Sauce can be refrigerated for up to two weeks. Remove from refrigerator and follow directions above.

---

*See Appendix B for more information on this product.

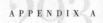

Tuna Salad on Cake

Serves 1

If you didn't prepare enough for leftovers the day before, this tuna recipe will do nicely for lunch or a late-night snack.

1	*unsalted rice cake*	*1*	*tablespoon chopped dill*
2	*ounces water-packed tuna*		*pickle*
	fish	*½*	*apple*
½	*tablespoon mayonnaise*		

Prepare the tuna salad, using the finely chopped dill pickles and mayonnaise. Spread it on the rice cake. Eat the apple for dessert!

Savory Baked Chicken

Serves 6
Prep time: 15 minutes
Cook time: 45 minutes

This recipe is ridiculously simple and was one of the first chicken recipes I taught my eight-year-old how to cook. The delicious gravy from the drippings will not upset your diet at all.

---

4 pounds chicken, cut into pieces
1¼ cups low-fat chicken broth
5–10 cloves garlic, minced
1 teaspoon salt substitute
1 teaspoon basil, fresh or dried

1 teaspoon parsley, fresh or dried
¼ teaspoon thyme, fresh or dried

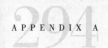

Prepare chicken for baking by removing the excess skin and visible fat. Place chicken in a baking dish, skin side up. Mix the rest of the ingredients together and spoon about one-third of the mixture over the chicken pieces, keeping the garlic and herbs on top of the chicken, if possible.

Bake at 400 degrees, uncovered, for about forty minutes or until done, basting periodically with the rest of the mixture until it is gone. Let the chicken brown nicely. When the chicken is done, remove the pieces from the pan and keep warm.

Defat the broth (see page 283). Pour into a skillet and boil gently until it thickens to the consistency of gravy. Serve the gravy in a separate bowl.

Meal-in-a-Flash Prep Plan
This meal is so simple that it really doesn't need a quicker idea. But in the morning before you leave for work, wash the chicken carefully and remove all the excess skin and visible fat. Dry with a paper towel and put in a food storage bag and seal tightly. Keep in the coldest part of the refrigerator.

Prepare the garlic now if you wish. Forty-five minutes before dinner is to be served, mix the broth with the herbs and garlic.

desserts

Orange Date Bars

Serves 24

You've been doing great . . . here is a treat! Warning: These cookies are a high-carbohydrate item you'll be tempted to snack on throughout the day. Include these cookies only in meals that are otherwise low in carbohydrates so you don't "carb out!"

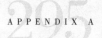
¼	cup butter	1	egg
1	cup spelt* or oat flour	½	teaspoon baking powder
⅓	cup honey	¼	teaspoon baking soda
1	teaspoon orange peel, finely shredded	½	cup walnuts, chopped
½	cup orange juice (with pulp if desired)	½	cup dates, pitted and chopped

In a food processor or mixer, process the butter for a few seconds. Add half the flour, the honey, orange peel, half of the orange juice, the egg, baking powder, and the baking soda. Beat until thoroughly mixed. Add the remaining flour and orange juice, and stir in the walnuts and dates. Spread the batter into an ungreased 11 x 7 x 1½-inch baking pan. Bake in a 350-degree oven about twenty-five minutes or until done.

Cool in the pan on a wire rack. Cut into bars. If you wish, you can substitute dried prunes for the dates. In that case, add ½ teaspoon ground cinnamon and a dash of cloves with the first flour.

Pumpkin Pie

Serves 6

This is our version of a traditional recipe, and you can't tell the difference. Satisfies your urge for something sweet, but if you balance it carefully with the rest of the meal, you'll stay in balance.

---

*See Appendix B for more information about this product.

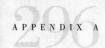
16	ounces cooked pumpkin	3	eggs
	(1 can)	1	cup goat or soy milk
⅓	cup sugar		pastry for single-crust pie
1	teaspoon ground cinnamon	8	fluid ounces light whipping
½	teaspoon ground ginger		cream
½	teaspoon ground nutmeg		

Mix together the pumpkin, sugar, and spices. Blend thoroughly. Add the eggs and beat thoroughly. Stir in the milk and mix well.

Pour into unbaked prepared pie shell and bake in a 375-degree oven for fifty minutes, or until a knife inserted near the center comes out clean. Serve with real whipped cream! Cover and chill to store.

Where to Find Specialty Food Items

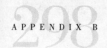

Black bean sauce: the gourmet section of your grocery store or your local Asian grocery.

Coconut milk: the gourmet section of your grocery store or your local Asian grocery store.

Corn pasta: most health food stores. You may substitute rice pasta if it's more convenient, but it's not as flavorful.

Curry paste: the gourmet section of your grocery store or your local Asian grocery store.

Fish sauce: the gourmet section of your grocery store or your local Asian grocery store.

Fresh herbs: the fresh-produce section of your grocery store. Rosemary and thyme can be frozen for up to two months. To store basil for a longer period of time, chop it finely and cover with olive oil. Keep in the refrigerator for four to five days, or freeze it for up to one month.

Fresh soba noodles: the produce section of your grocery store.

Hot chili paste: the specialty section of your grocery store.

Hoisin sauce: the Asian section of your grocery store or in an Asian grocery store.

Jicama: a vegetable found in the fresh produce section of most grocery stores.

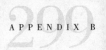

Mesclun mix: This prepackaged blend of different types of greens is in the fresh-produce section.

Red miso: the Asian section of your grocery store or in an Asian grocery store.

Sherry vinegar: the gourmet or condiment section of your grocery store.

Spelt flour: Because wheat is a highly allergenic food, we prefer to eliminate all wheat products. Spelt flour is not as problematic for most people and can be purchased in most health food stores. You may also use barley or oat flour if you prefer. If you use rice flour, you may need to reduce the amount of flour in a recipe.

Wasabi powder: the specialty section of your local grocery store.

Reference
Section

C

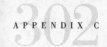

Your local health food and supplement store, or your local General Nutrition Center (GNC) should be able to provide you with most products I have recommended. For those products not available locally or through retail outlets, contact:

Eat Away
Enique International
101 E. 8th St., Suite 120, Vancouver, WA 98660
800-288-2800

Meal Replacement Bars or Dietary Supplements
The Health Haus, Inc.
800-652-2765

The Nutritionist Series products
The Health Haus, Inc.
800-652-2765

Allergy Testing and Hair Analysis
The Natural Physician Center
503-526-8600

American Phytotherapy Research Laboratory
P.O. Box 372
Lehi, UT 84043
801-572-7666

Nature's Secret products
800-297-3273

1. L. Kathleen Mahan and Marian Arlin, *Krause's Food, Nutrition & Diet Therapy* (Philadelphia: W. B. Saunders, 1992), 316.

2. Ibid.

3. "The Number of Overweight Youths Doubled in the Past Decade, New Study Says," *Nutrition Week* 25, no. 38 (6 October 1995): 1.

4. Aviva Must, Ph.D. et al., "Long-Term Morbidity and Mortality of Overweight Adolescents: A Follow-up of the Harvard Growth Study of 1922–1935," *New England Journal of Medicine* (5 November 1992): 1350–55; cited in *Clinical Pearls* (1992): 372.

5. Peter N. Benotti and R. Armour Forse, "The Role of Gastric Surgery in the Multi-Disciplinary Management of Severe Obesity," *American Journal of Surgery* 169, no. 3 (March 1995): 361; Mahan and Arlin, *Krause's Food, Nutrition & Diet Therapy*, 316.

6. "It's Time to Regulate the Diet Industry: We Need an Accrediting Agency That Would Protect Patients and Make Doctors' Jobs Easier As Well," *Medical Economics* (8 March 1993): 23–30; cited in *Clinical Pearls* (1993): 289; Mara Bovsum, "The Diet Dilemma," *Medical World News* (May 1992): 17–25; cited in *Clinical Pearls* (1992): 373.

7. Benotti, "The Role of Gastric Surgery," p. 361.

8. Steven Shepherd, *Executive Health Report* 24, no. 7 (April 1988): 7.

9. Sirpa Sarlio-Lahteenkorva, Albert Stunkard, and Aila Rissanen, "Psychosocial Factors and Quality of Life In Obesity," *International Journal of Obesity* 19, supplement 6 (1995): S1–S5.

10. Bovsum, pp. 17–25.

11. Frank Minirth, M.D., Dr. Paul Meier, Dr. Robert Hemfelt, and Dr. Sharon Sneed, *Love Hunger Weight-Loss Workbook* (Nashville: Thomas Nelson, 1991), p. 7.

12. James Groff, Sareen Gropper, and Sara M. Hunt, *Advanced Nutrition and Human Metabolism* (Minneapolis/St. Paul: West, 1995), pp. 443–44.

chapter two: five common strategies to avoid

1. John D. Cunningham, *Human Biology* (New York: Harper & Row, 1989), p. 247.

2. *American Heritage Illustrated Encyclopedic Dictionary*, 1987 ed., s.v. "Homeostasis."

3. L. Kathleen Mahan and Marian Arlin, *Krause's Food, Nutrition and Diet Therapy* (Philadelphia: W. B. Saunders, 1992), p. 318.

4. "Eat More to Lose More (Higher Metabolism Burns More Calories)," *The Edell Health Letter* 12, no. 2 (February 1993): 1(1).

5. V. George, "Small Eaters and Large Eaters," *Nutrition Research Newsletter* 8, no. 4 (April 1989): 44(10).

6. Paula Derrow, *Weight Watchers Magazine* (July 1993): 14 (3).

7. G. F. Adami, P. Gandolfo, A. Compostano, F. Coechi, B. Bauer, and N. Scorpinaro, "Obese Binge Eaters: Metabolic Characteristics, Energy Expenditure and Dieting," *Psychological Medicine* 25 (1995): 195–98; Sheila Specker, Martina deZwaah, Nancy Raymond, and James Mitchell, "Psychopathology in Subgroups of Obese Women With and Without Binge Eating Disorder," *Comprehensive Psychiatry* 35, no. 3 (May/June 1994): 185–90.

8. Timothy D. Brewerton, "Toward a Unified Theory of Serotonin Dysregulation in Eating and Related Disorders," *Psychoneuroendocrinology* 20, no. 6 (1995): 561–90.

9. Specker et al. "Psychopathology in Subgroups of Obese Women," 187.

10. Sheila Specker, Sylvia T. Lae, and Marilyn Carroll, "Food Deprivation History and Cocaine Self-Administration: An Animal Model of Binge Eating," *Pharmacology Biochemistry and Behavior* 48, no. 4 (1994): 1025–29; Kenneth D. Carr and Vassiliki Papadouka, "The Role of Multiple Opioid Receptors in the Potentiation of Reward by Food Restriction," *Brain Research* 639 (1994): 253–60.

11. Janet Polivy, Sharon Zeitlin, C. Peter Herman, and A. Lynne Beal, "Food Restriction and Binge Eating: A Study of Former Prisoners of War," *Journal of Abnormal Psychology* 103, no. 2 (1994): 409–11.

12. A. R. Spalter, H. E. Gwirtsman, M. A. Demitrack, and P. W. Gold, "Thyroid Function in Bulimia Nervosa," *Biological Psychiatry* 33, no. 6 (15 March 1993): 408–14.

13. D. C. Jimerson, M. D. Lesem, W. H. Kaye, and T. D. Brewerton, "Low Serotonin and Dopamine Metabolite Concentrations in Cerebrospinal Fluid from Bulimic Patients with Frequent Binge Episodes," *Archives of General Psychiatry* 49, no. 2 (February 1992): 132–38.

14. Brewerton, p. 569.

15. David G. Schlundt, James O. Hill, Tracy Sbrocco, Jamie Pope-Cordle, and Teresa Sharp, "The Role of Breakfast in the Treatment of Obesity: A Randomized Clinical Trial," *American Journal of Clinical Nutrition* 55 (1992): 645–51.

16. Thomas A. Wadden, Gary D. Foster, and Kathleen A. Letizia, "One-Year Behavioral Treatment of Obesity: Comparison of Moderate and Severe Caloric Restriction and the Effects of Weight Maintenance Therapy," *Journal of Consulting and Clinical Psychology* 62, no. 1 (1994): 165–71.

17. Neal Barnard, M.D., *Eat Right Live Longer* (New York: Harmony Books, 1995), p. 295.

18. Douglas B. White, Bin He, Roger G. Dean, and Roy J. Martin, "Low Protein Diets Increase Neuropeptide Y Gene Expression in the Basomedial Hypothalamus of Rats," *Journal of Nutrition* 124, no. 8 (August 1994): 1152–59.

19. Ronald F. Schmid, N.D., *Native Nutrition* (Rochester, VT: Healing Arts Press, 1994), p. 155. Arachidonic acid is a pro-inflammatory, pro-weight-gain fatty acid.

20. Ibid., p. 155.

21. Corinne T. Netzer, *The Complete Book of Food Counts* (New York: Dell, 1991).

22. Ann Louise Gittleman, M.S., with J. Maxwell Desgrey, *Beyond Pritikin* (New York: Bantam, 1988), pp. 10–11.

23. Schmid, p. 88.

24. Udo Erasmus, *Fats and Oils* (Vancouver, B.C.: Alive Books, 1986), p. 35.

25. Mahan and Arlin, p. 317.

26. Robert Erdmann, Ph.D., and Meririon Jones, *Fats That Can Save Your Life: The Critical Role of Fats and Oils in Health and Disease* (Encinitas, CA: Progressive Health Publishing, 1995), pp. 61–62.

27. Erasmus, p. 41.

28. Barry Sears, Ph.D., *The Zone* (New York: HarperCollins, 1995), pp. 19–20.

29. Larry S. Hobbs, "Ephedrine + Caffeine = The Ideal Diet Pill," *Townsend Letter for Doctors* (June 1996): 66–67.

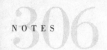

1. Daniel Mowrey, Ph.D., *Fat Management! The Thermogenic Factor* (Lehi, UT: Victory Publications, 1994), p. 108.

2. B. Jeanrenaud, "Hyperinsulinemia in Obesity Syndromes: Its Metabolic Consequences and Possible Etiology," *Metabolism* 27, supplement 2 (December 1978): 1881–92.

3. P. U. Dubuc, "The Development of Obesity, Hyperinsulinemia, and Hyperglycemia in Ob/OB Mice," *Metabolism* 25 (December 1976): 1567–74.

4. Celia Garcia-Martinez, Francisca J. Lopez-Soriano, and Josep M. Argiles, "Intestinal Glucose Absorption Is Lower in Obese Than in Lean Zucker Rats," *Journal of Nutrition* 123, no. 6 (June 1993): 1062.

5. Thomas J. Lauterio, J. Preston Bond, and Edward A. Ulmar, "Development and Characterization of a Purified Diet to Identify Obesity-Susceptible and Resistant Rat Populations," *Journal of Nutrition* 124, no. 11 (November 1994): 2132.

6. U.S. Department of Commerce, *Statistical Abstract of the United States* (Washington, D.C.: GPO, 1995), p. 148.

7. J. A. Higgins, Janette C. Brand Miller, and Gareth J. Denyer, "Development of Insulin Resistance in the Rat Is Dependent on the Rate of Glucose Absorption from the Diet," *Journal of Nutrition* 126, no. 3 (March 1996): 596–602.

8. R. J. Barnard, J. F. Youngren, and D. A. Martin, "Diet, Not Aging, Causes Skeletal Muscle Insulin Resistance," *Gerontology* 41, no. 4 (1995): 205–11.

9. S. M. Virtanen, J. Sau Kkohen, E. Savilahti, K. Ylonen, L. Rasanen, P. Aro, Miknip, J. Tuomilehto, and H. K. Akerblom, "Diet, Cow's Milk Protein Antibodies and the Risk of IDDM in Finnish Children," *Diabetologia* 37, no. 4 (April 1994): 381–87; Virtanen et al., "Dietary Factors in the Aetiology of Diabetes," *Annals of Medicine* 26, no. 6 (December 1994): 469–78.

10. D. B. West, C. N. Boozer, D. L. Moody, and R. L. Atkinson, "Dietary Obesity in Nine Inbred Mouse Strains," *American Journal of Physiology* 262, no. 6 (2) (June 1992): R1025–32.

11. Ben Greenstein, *Endocrinology at a Glance* (London: Blackwell Science, 1994), p. 8.

1. Gerard J. Tortora and Sandrea Reynolds Grabowski, *Principles of Anatomy and Physiology* (New York: HarperCollins College Publishers, 1993), p. 537.

2. Francis S. Greenspan and John D. Baxter, *Basic and Clinical Endocrinology* (Norwalk, CT: Appleton & Lange, 1994), p. 175.

3. Ibid., p. 186.

4. W. M. Wiersinga, "Subclinical Hypothyroidism and Hyperthyroidism: Prevalence in Clinical Relevance," *Netherlands Journal of Medicine* 46 (1995): 197–204; cited in *Clinical Pearls* (1995): 266.

5. Broda O. Barnes, M.D., and Lawrence Galton, *Hypothyroidism: The Unsuspected Illness* (New York: Harper & Row, 1976), pp. 45–47.

6. Telephone interview with Denis Wilson, M.D. (17 July 1996), Vancouver, Washington.

7. W. P. Pimenta et al., "The Assessment of Zinc Status by the Zinc Tolerance Test and Thyroid Disease," *Trace Elements in Medicine* 9, no. 1 (1992): 34–37; cited in *Clinical Pearls* (1992): 443.

8. Norman Campbell, M.D., "Ferrous Sulfate Reduces Thyroxine Efficacy in Patients with Hypothyroidism," *Annals of Internal Medicine* 117, no. 12 (15 December 1992): 1010–13; cited in *Clinical Pearls* (1992).

9. Elson M. Haas, M.D., *Staying Healthy with Nutrition* (Berkeley, CA: Celestial Arts, 1992), pp. 194–95.

10. Ross I. McDougall, *Thyroid Disease in Clinical Practice* (New York: Oxford University Press, 1992), pp. 164–65.

11. Haas, p. 196.

12. Ibid., p. 196.

13. L. A. McKeown, "Nuclear Cleanups Will Cost Billions," *Medical Tribune* 3 (28 January 1993); cited in *Clinical Pearls* (1993): 142.

14. Stephen E. Langer, M.D., and James F. Scheer, *Solved: The Riddle of Illness* (New Canaan, CT: Keats, 1995), pp. 39–41.

15. Ibid., pp. 102–3.

16. National Task Force on the Prevention and Treatment of Obesity, "Weight Cycling," *JAMA* 272, no. 15 (19 October 1994): 1201.

17. K. D. D. Brownell and J. Rodin, "Medical, Metabolic, and Psychological Effects of Weight Cycling," *Archives of Internal Medicine* 154 (27 June 1994): 1326.

18. Ibid., pp. 1325–30.

19. Normal Marine, M.D., et al., "Dietary Restriction on Serum Thyroid Hormone Levels," *The American Journal of Medical Sciences* 301 (May 1991): 310–13; cited in *Clinical Pearls* (1991): 334.

20. Diana M. Gonzales-Pacheco, William Buss, Kathleen M. Koehler, William Woodridge, and Seymour Alpert, "Energy Restriction Reduces Metabolic Rate in Adult Male Fisher-344 Rats," *Journal of Nutrition* 123, no. 1 (January 1993): 90.

21. Malcolm H. Wheeler and John H. Lazarus, *Diseases of the Thyroid* (London: Chapman & Hall, 1994), p. 274.

22. Ibid., p. 276.

23. M. J. Soares, R. N. Kulkarni, L. S. Diers, M. Vaz, and P. S. Shetty, "Energy Supplementation Reverses Changes in the Basal Metabolic Rates of Chronically Undernourished Individuals," *British Journal of Nutrition* 68 (1992): 593–602.

chapter five: fat, frustrated, forty, and female

1. Ben Greenstein, *Endocrinology at a Glance* (London: Blackwell Science, 1994), p. 63.

2. Kenneth L. Becker et al., *Principles and Practice of Endocrinology and Metabolism,* (Philadelphia: Lippincott, 1990), p. 897.

3. Greenstein, p. 50.

4. Daniel Mowrey, Ph.D., *Fat Management! The Thermogenic Factor* (Lehi, UT: Victory Publications, 1994), p. 177.

5. David Watts, Ph.D., "The Nutritional Relationships of Copper," *Trace Elements* 208 (1995): 103–4.

6. David Watts, Ph.D., *Trace Elements and Other Essential Nutrients: Clinical Application of Tissue Mineral Analysis* (Dallas, TX: Trace Elements, Inc., 1995), pp. 84–85.

7. Greenstein, p. 23.

8. James W. Long, M.D., *The Essential Guide to Prescription Drugs, 1992* (New York: Harper Perennial, 1992), p. 491.

9. Ann Louise Gittleman, M.D., *Super Nutrition for Menopause* (New York: Pocket Books, 1993), pp. 26–27.

10. Telephone interview with Calvin Ezrin, M.D., 12 July 1995, Vancouver, Washington.

11. David V. Schapira et al., "Abdominal Obesity and Breast Cancer Risk," *Annals of Internal Medicine* 112, no. 3 (1 February 1990): 182(5); as cited in *Clinical Pearls* (1990): 83.

chapter six: squabbling sisters

1. Patsy Bostick Reed, *Nutrition: An Applied Science* (St. Paul: West, 1980), p. 22.

2. Jean-Pierre Flatt, "Use and Storage of Carbohydrate and Fat," *American Journal of Clinical Nutrition* 61 (Suppl.) (1995): 9525–95.

3. Ben Greenstein, *Endocrinology at a Glance* (London: Blackwell Science, 1994), p. 82.

4. Francis S. Greenspan and John D. Baxter, *Basic and Clinical Endocrinology* (Norwalk, CT: Appleton & Lange, 1994), pp. 576–77.

5. Reed, p. 35.

6. Ibid., p. 27.

7. Greenspan and Baxter, p. 576.

8. Ibid., p. 576.

9. Ibid., p. 577.

10. Barry Sears, Ph.D., *In the Zone* (New York: HarperCollins, 1995), p. 30.

11. Daniel Mowrey, Ph.D., *Fat Management! The Thermogenic Factor* (Lehi, UT: Victory Publications, 1994), p. 164.

12. Jing Ju et al., "Dietary (N-3) Polyunsaturated Fatty Acids Improve Adipocyte Insulin Action and Glucose Metabolism in Insulin-Resistant Rats: Relation to Membrane Fatty Acids," *Journal of Nutrition* 126, no. 8 (August 1996): 1953.

13. Jeffrey Moss, D.D.S., "Hyperinsulinemia and Insulin Resistance—A Missing Link in Obesity and Cardiovascular Disease," *The Townsend Letter for Doctors* 99 (April 1996).

14. Greenspan and Baxter, p. 576.

15. Frank Murray, *The Big Family Guide to All the Minerals* (New Canaan, CT: Keats, 1995), pp. 243–44.

16. Reed, p. 376.

17. L. Kathleen Mahan and Marian Arlin, *Krause's Food, Nutrition and Diet Therapy* (Philadelphia: W. B. Saunders, 1992), p. 131.

18. Murray, p. 245.

19. D. Baly et al., "Effect of Manganese Deficiency on Insulin Binding, Glucose Transport, and Metabolism in Rat Adipocytes," *Journal of Nutrition* 120 (1990): 1075–79; cited in Frank Murray, *The Big Family Guide to All the Minerals.*

20. Baly et al., p. 1078.

21. Murray, p. 324.

22. Mahan and Arlin, p. 136.

23. Reed, p. 378.

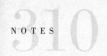
24. Dallas Clouatre, Ph.D., *Getting Lean with Anti-Fat Nutrients* (San Francisco: Pax Publishing, 1993), p. 22.

25. C. Carl Pfeiffer, Ph.D., M.D., *Mental and Elemental Nutrients* (New Canaan, CT: Keats, 1975), p. 24.

26. Mildred S. Seelig, M.D., M.P.H., F.A.C.N., *Magnesium Deficiency in the Pathogenesis of Disease* (New York: Plenum Medical Book Company, 1980), p. 262.

27. J. Ishizuka et al., "In Vitro Relationship Between Magnesium and Insulin Secretion," *Magnesium Research* 7, no. 1 (March 1994): 17–22; M. Murakami, J. Ishizuka, S. Sumi, G. A. Nichols, C. W. Cooper, C. M. Townsend, Jr., and J. C. Thompson, "Role of Extracellular Magnesium in Insulin Secretion From Rat Insulinoma Cells," *Proceedings of the Society for Experimental Biology and Medicine* 200, no. 4 (September 1992): 490–94.

28. Richard N. Podell, M.D., and William Proctor, *The G-Index Diet: The Missing Link That Makes Permanent Weight Loss Possible* (New York: Warner Books, 1993), p. 4.

chapter seven: the good news

1. "Stress and the Heart: Mechanisms, Measurement and Management," *Postgraduate Medicine* 92, no. 5 (October 1992): 237–48.

2. Press Release, David Brett Wasser, Media Director, Physician's Committee for Responsible Medicine (25 January 1996).

3. "Olestra and Frito-Lay," *Nutrition Week* (7 June 1996): 7; cited in *Clinical Pearls* (1996): 164.

4. H. L. Newbold, M.D., *Dr. Newbold's Type A, Type B Weight Loss Book* (New Canaan, CT: Keats, 1991).

Carol is available to guest-lecture to professionals working with weight-challenged individuals, or on other topics such as depression, attention deficit hyperactivity disorder, fibromyalgia, recovery from surgery/illness, and PMS/menopause.

if you have questions

Carol would love to hear from her readers about their experiences on the No Fault/No Fat program, and answer any questions they may have.

Please feel free to write her:

c/o The Health Haus Inc.
101 E. 8th St. #250
Vancouver, WA 98660

index

about the authors

Carol Simontacchi is CEO of the Health Haus Inc., a chain of health and nutrition stores; host of a daily radio talk show now in its sixth year; and author of books, training courses, and the Natural Balance Weight Management Program. Carol is also the founder of The Natural Physician Center in Beaverton, Oregon. A graduate of the National Institute for Nutritional Education in Aurora, Colorado, she earned her Master of Science in Social Science from Columbia Pacific University. Carol served as President of the Society for Certified Nutritionists from 1991 to 1993 and continues her involvement as she serves on the board of directors. As an active member of the National Nutritional Foods Association, Carol serves as Chair of the Education Committee. She is a Certified Clinical Nutritionist through the International and American Associations of Clinical Nutritionists.

She lives in Vancouver, Washington, with her husband and four young daughters.

Margaret (Meg) West is a graduate of the California Culinary Academy. She has worked at many nationally renowned restaurants, including Chez Panisse. She is now working with The Natural Physician Center, designing menu programs for nutritionally challenged clients and is involved with two other books on weight loss and other health issues. She is married and the mother of two young sons.